Contents

KU-200-014

Acknowledgements

I would like to express my gratitude to Mr Hackman, Consultant Obstetrician and Gynaecologist at Peterborough Maternity Unit for introducing me to ultrasound, and to all of my colleagues in ultrasound, in particular Geraldine Ward.

Lastly, I would like to thank my husband John and my family for their continuing support.

Ultrasound
for
Midwives
A Guide for Midwives and other Health Professionals

Jean Proud SRN, SCM, MTD

Books for Midwives Press
Books for Midwives Press is a joint publishing venture
between The Royal College of Midwives and
Haigh & Hochland Publications Ltd

Published by Books for Midwives Press, 174a Ashley Road, Hale, Cheshire, WA15 9SF, England

©1994, Jean Proud

First edition

ISBN 1-898507-03-1

British Library Cataloguing in Publication Data
A catalogue record for this book is available from the British Library

Printed in Great Britain by RAP Ltd

CHAPTER 1

Basic Technology

"New technology should not be widely used before it has been fully evaluated, but there is considerable doubt whether this is the case in respect of current practice of ultrasonography" wrote Marian Hall, MD (Consultant Obstetrician and Gynaecologist at Aberdeen Royal Infirmary) in the British Medical Journal in 1991. Yet ultrasound scanning is now an integral part of ante-natal care in Great Britain today. Most women are offered a scan at some stage of their pregnancy, usually in the first or second trimester.

What then is this technology?

Ultrasound is sound waves produced at a very high frequency. Bats use it in navigation. The means to detect and use it were discovered as long ago as 1880.

The technology of ultrasound was developed following the loss of the Titanic and used extensively in the two world wars to track and destroy submarines. Sound waves bounce off solid objects, and the echoes produced build up a picture of the object.

In the 1950s Professor Iain Donald, then Regius Professor of Midwifery at Glasgow University, pioneered its use in obstetrics. At first, because of the need to transmit the sound waves through water to obtain an adequate image, he submerged his subjects in a large cylindrical water bath. Subsequently, filling the urinary bladder acted as the fluid medium through which he created a suitable window.

In the early days, the images were very black and white and only the outline of the major structures could be seen. It was not until the 1970s that Professor Wells in Bristol developed grey scale which enabled various tissues to be differentiated and characterised. This tissue characterisation is brought about by the way the tissues react to the sound waves. The different textures produce a variety of patterns. In this way, the character of an individual tissue is recognised. This characterisation is widely used both in the establishment of the normal pattern of a certain organ, and also in enabling the recognition of any abnormal patterns which denote the presence of any abnormality or disease.

In the early days of diagnostic ultrasound the machines were large and unwieldy and the pictures static, although beautifully clear. Large gantries were needed which were difficult to manoeuvre, especially with the speed and agility needed to examine the moving fetus. Ultrasound examination became a lot easier when real-time scanning was invented. Real-time scanners are the machines which are used today. Moving pictures can be seen, enabling fetal movement, cardiac activity and behavioural patterns to be studied.

More recently Doppler machines, which enable the volume of moving liquids, for example blood, to be estimated, have become incorporated into real-time scanners. They can also be used independently, as part of the screening programme in the larger centres.

How is Ultrasound Produced?

The principal of ultrasound is sound, produced by a type of electric gong at a high pitch, and transmitted in a narrow beam. The piece of equipment involved is known as a transducer or probe. It changes electrical energy into sound and back again.

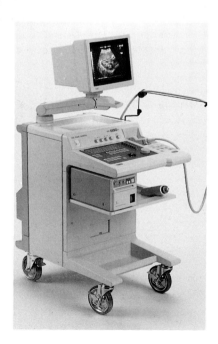

Fig. 1.1 Real-time ultrasound machine

How does Ultrasound Work?

The transducer is placed on the part to be scanned, and sound waves are passed into the body. As a structure is encountered, a small amount of sound is reflected back. This echo is detected electronically and transmitted onto the screen as a dot. The amount of sound reflected from each organ varies according to the type of tissue encountered. The image produced on the screen thus varies in texture and shades of grey, from black (which denotes a fluid) to white (which denotes a dense structure, for example, bone).

Transducers

There are various types of transducers which can basically be divided into two main groups. The first group are *sector scanners* which are mechanical. They produce a sector shaped image on the screen. This produces a whirring sound which can be heard when the machine is in use.

There are two types of mechanical scanners. In one type, a single crystal oscillates backwards and forwards through an angle of 90 degrees. The other type has three or four crystals placed on a wheel which rotates rapidly. Both mechanisms are suspended in an oil medium at the scanner head which is rounded, small, light and easy to hold. It can be very useful for angling into the nooks and crannies of the anatomy, for example, behind the symphysis to examine the pelvic organs, or through the anterior fontanelle of the neonatal skull to examine the contents.

Sector scanners are mainly used for abdominal scanning, to visualise a small section of the anatomy through a small window. Due to this small window they are not so useful for examination of the developing fetus in the second or the third trimesters.

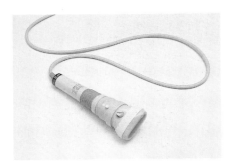

Fig. 1.2 Illustration of a sector head

The second type are *electronic scanners* or *linear* or *curvilinear transducers*. They have a crystal system which is divided into many parts on a line along the length of the transducer. These crystals number anything from 100-600. They fire off electrical energy in small groups in rapid succession along the length of the transducer. The advantage of this type of transducer is that there is a wide field of view directly from the abdominal surface. The sonographer can usually get quite a clear view for a considerable depth by altering the resolution using a selector system. The transducers are quite long, about 9 or 10 inches. They can be difficult to manipulate in the transverse plane, when trying to scan a thin woman between the iliac crests. A more recent development, the curved linear transducer gives a long, slightly sectional image. These transducers have become popular in obstetric scanning because one can examine the fetus in detail. The resolution is usually good to a considerable depth, and they are easier to manipulate than the straight linear probe. Both the straight and the curvilinear transducers are inclined to be heavier than the sector probes, because of their multicrystal make up. This necessitates a great many electrical wires being wound round together in what becomes quite a thick cable.

In recent years, vaginal scanning has become the method of choice in the first trimester of pregnancy, and for gynaecological examinations. It is particularly useful for women undergoing fertility investigations.

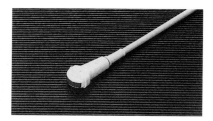

Fig. 1.3 Illustration of curvilinear pr obe

Vaginal ultrasound has been found to be advantageous because of the proximity of the transducer to the structures it visualises. It is particularly useful when investigating the follicular development within the ovary. The probes can be electrical or mechanical, but the electrical variety are usually preferred because they are more reliable. Mechanical systems can break. Whatever type of transducer is used, the image received and portrayed on the screen conventionally has the maternal bladder and the symphysis to the right, and the fundus or the xiphistemum to the left, in the longitudinal plane. If this is adhered to, mistakes in diagnosis are less likely to occur, for example, placenta praevia will not be mistaken for a fundally situated placenta!

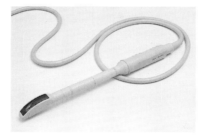

Fig. 1.4 Illustration of a vaginal probe

Doppler Ultrasound

Many women, especially in larger centres, now undergo further investigations of measurement of blood flow through the maternal and/or the fetal vessels. This necessitates the use of Doppler equipment. One form of Doppler equipment familiar to most doctors and midwives is the type used to listen to the fetal heart. The sound waves on reception are amplified so that they can be heard. The same sort of device is used to monitor the blood flow wave forms in the uterine, placental and fetal vessels. In most machines it is not possible to see the vessel. If this is required, a duplex scanner, or a combined system is needed.

One problem with duplex scanners is that the amount of ultrasound energy is greater than that used in diagnostic ultrasound, or in the conventional Doppler machines. Colour Doppler is now a feature that can aid clinicians in identifying flow towards, and away from, the fields examined. This has particular significance for diagnosis and identification of tumours.

Calibration

A feature of all types of scanner is the facility for calibration. As one of the principle uses is measurement of the fetus for the purpose of estimating gestational age, or assessing growth patterns, it is essential that these measurements are accurate. Incorporated into the computer soft-ware is a facility for calculating the size of the structures visualised, or the blood velocity within a particular vessel. This facility has become very sophisticated. Linear measurements, circumferences and areas can be obtained at the touch of a button, after a series of markers have been positioned correctly. Similarly, blood velocity wave forms can be studied.

5

Keeping accurate records

Recording the information obtained is vitally important. Midwives have a statutory duty to keep records of all their examinations of pregnant woman (*Midwives Rules, 1993*)

Clear records not only include written reports of examinations. Video recordings, and/or the facility to take Polaroid photographs, are incorporated within most ultrasound systems. Whether these are used for every woman as a matter of routine, or for the identification or recording of an abnormality, the legal implications must be considered. When recording abnormalities so that evidence can be submitted, or a second opinion obtained, there are medico-legal considerations to be taken into account. A third party could be brought in to pass an opinion if a recording is made. If there is no recording, this cannot happen. If a recording is made it is part of the woman's records and should be treated in the same way as written records, the obligation being to retain it for 25 years (*Midwives Rules, 1993*). Such recordings are invalid if there is no name or date recorded on them.

This has been a very brief resumé of the technology to give the reader an introduction to what is the main purpose of this book; an understanding of a) the potential of diagnostic ultrasound in obstetrics, b) its interpretation, and c) some of the constraints.

No technology should be used until it has been deemed to be safe. The debate on the safety of ultrasound, particularly with regard to diagnostic ultrasound is discussed in the next chapter.

Whether the technology has been properly evaluated is debatable. Perhaps this book will help practitioners of midwifery and obstetrics to decide for themselves. The question about its frequent, and sometimes indiscriminate use during pregnancy needs to be addressed by all professionals. Before any scan the question to be considered is: Is this scan really necessary?

CHAPTER 2

Safety Issues

Professor Peter Wells, (Dept. of Medical Physics, Bristol General Hospital), in his presidential address to the British Institute of Radiology on May 25th 1986, said: *"The prudent use of ultrasound diagnosis depends on its being used cautiously, carefully, circumspectly, judiciously, sensibly, and wisely: like other technologies in medicine, diagnostic ultrasound is a resource which should be used with skill and good judgement"* (Wells, 1987a).

When considering if ultrasound is safe, the following questions need to be asked:-
1) Is the technology safe?
2) Is the use of the technology safe?
3) Can one rely on the information obtained when using it?
4) Is the operator of the technology trained sufficiently to use it, so that a correct interpretation of the data obtained can be given? and
5) Is the operator working within the realm of safe practice?

1)Is the technology safe?
Since the inception of the use of ultrasound in medicine, studies have been undertaken to look for potential damaging effects. The experiments that have been carried out have been done, in the main, by independent investigators, many of whom have had little knowledge of the biology or the physics they have been investigating *(Wells, 1987b)*. So far diagnostic ultrasound, or the levels of ultrasound used for diagnostic purposes, have not produced any indications to suggest that it is not safe to use for that purpose.

One cannot prove safety, however, by showing negative results. There is only an absence of any evidence of a confirmed hazard. The enthusiasm of scientists and manufacturers in the 1970s and 80s to produce machines that gave better and clearer pictures meant that output levels of ultrasound rose accordingly.

In 1984 a certain amount of publicity about the safety of diagnostic ultrasound called into question its routine use in obstetrics. This followed disturbing reports from a number of studies suggesting the possibility of its biological effects and possible hazards (*Kremkau 1983; Liebeskind et al, 1979; MacIntosh & Davey 1970 & 1972; Testart et al, 1982)*. The Scientific Advisory Committee of the Royal College of Obstetricians and Gynaecologists set up a working party to advise on the advantages and disadvantages of routine ultrasound examination in pregnancy. At that time 64% of the 191 health districts in England offered a routine scan to all mothers. Of the remaining 36%, 22% offered a routine scan to a proportion of the women in their care. This was usually a reflection of the policies of the different consultants. Taking into account the fact that most of the others were offered a scan for some reason, that is they were selectively, as opposed to routinely, scanned, it was estimated that some 85% of women had a scan sometime in their pregnancy. In Germany and Sweden it was almost 100% (R.C.O.G., 1984).

The working party reviewed the literature that had been produced and came up with some recommendations. They did not see a need to change the practice of routinely scanning women in the second trimester of pregnancy, but identified the need for a large well planned prospective study. This was intended to determine the extent of the benefits of routine scanning over selective scanning for obstetric or medical indications.

(This is discussed further in Chapter 3)

The working party felt that, although written consent to ultrasound examination was not necessary, women should be given a written explanation of the reasons why the procedure was recommended. Not only that, but also the sonographer should make sure that women have read and understood it, before proceeding with the examination.

To the author's knowledge very few women do receive a written explanation of the reasons why their scan is thought to be necessary. More often than not they are presented with a form to take along to the imaging department at the hospital, having had very little counselling regarding the nature of the investigation from either midwives or medical clinicians.

Questions of training in the technique of ultrasound, supervision and the positioning of the equipment were addressed by the working party. The final recommendation stated that the beam intensities of the machines should be standardised and that manufacturers should be required to publicise the maximum intensity values. These values should be kept to the minimum amount to enable a satisfactory image to be obtained. They also suggested that a government agency be appointed to 'spot' check the power output levels of the machines used for diagnostic purposes. *(R.C.O.G., 1984)*

Since 1984 acoustic output levels of ultrasound energy used by machines intended for diagnostic purposes have been standardised. The levels are published in the machine manuals and must be within the safety limits agreed by the watchdog bodies. The levels are expressed in values of spatial peak intensity averaged over time (SPTA). The American Institute of Ultrasound in Medicine recommended that this should be less than 100mW/cm2. The British Medical Ultrasound Society agreed to adopt the same values.

The National Institutes of Health Consensus Development Conference held in the same year in Bethesda U.S.A. also studied the then current practice of ultrasound and issued their report. Unlike their British counterparts they came to the conclusion that *"It is recommended that the indications for and limitations in the use of ultrasound should be: ultrasound scanning in pregnancy should be performed for a specific medical indication; other usage should be discouraged; mothers should be informed of clinical reasons for scanning and the benefit/risk factor; minimum training requirements for sonography should be established; and further studies on bioeffects should be carried out"(Wells, 1987b)*

Also in 1984, the Diagnostic Methods Committee of the British Institute of Radiology recommended that a working party be set up to examine specifically *"the controversy relating to the safety of diagnostic ultrasound"*. The working group was to *"review the scientific evidence"*. This working group limited its considerations to that alone. They did not address the issue of use of the technology.

The conclusion was *"There is no reason to suspect that any hazard exists"*. The report itself is published by the British Institute of Radiology *(Wells, 1987b)*. The working party again reviewed the literature published regarding the biological effects of ultrasound at levels used for diagnostic purposes and the human epidemiological studies. It also examined the exposure conditions that were used at that time in diagnostic ultrasound.

The Biological Effects of Ultrasound

Energy produces heat. Ultrasound energy is no exception. As ultrasound energy passes through tissue, heat is produced. It is precisely because of this that physiotherapists use it for treating the perineum in the post-natal period. The levels of energy used by them are much greater than that used for diagnostic purposes. The rise in temperature in the tissues during a diagnostic investigation has been shown to be no different from the normal diurnal variation over a twenty-four hour period which is one degree Celsius. This is, therefore, probably harmless *(Kremkau 1983)*. As power is increased to the range used by physiotherapists, this temperature rises. Some pulsed Doppler machines, which do have a greater output of energy, should therefore be used very cautiously.

Another potential problem is cavitation, or the formation of gas bubbles in the tissues, which grow in certain conditions and then burst. This has the potential of generating very high temperatures. Oscillation of these bubbles could cause damage to the cells and the cell membrane. This phenomenon has been observed in plants *(Haar & Daniels, 1981 & Haar et al, 1982)*. Levels used in diagnostic ultrasound are lower than those used in these experiments. Cavitation, however, is not thought to be a problem at the levels of output used for diagnostic purposes *(Evans, 1992)*.

MacIntosh and Davey *(1970 & 1972)*, reported that they had observed damage to chromosomes induced by diagnostic levels of ultrasound. This startling revelation instigated a series of studies attempting to duplicate the findings. They were performed under a variety of conditions, using a variety of frequencies. The fear was that not only might the chromosomes be damaged, but that the technique might cause mutations leading to the development of tumours. The power used ranged from diagnostic to therapeutic levels, but no evidence was found to suggest the occurrence of change. But as Peter Wells *(1977)* pointed out , if chromosome damage were to occur, the most likely outcome would be death of the cell.

Sister chromatid exchange (i.e. portions of the two chromatids exchange) has also been reported *(Liebeskind et al, 1979)*. There is little evidence to suggest that this is of any significance. Most of the experiments have been carried out on animal tissue or in vitro. Human studies are few, but the relationship between ultrasound levels and malignancy has been examined by Kinnear, Wilson & Waterhouse in 1984, and also by Cartwright et al, in 1984. The results were reassuring, but it was recognised that a great many more long term studies needed to be carried out.

Among the epidemiological studies that have been carried out is one by Stark et al *(1984)* who attempted to follow up children who had been exposed to ultrasound in utero. No problems were found for the majority, although concern was raised about dyslexia which seemed to have an association with exposure to ultrasound in utero. However, this was inconclusive. More recent studies have indicated similar findings. A Norwegian study examined 2161 children of women who took part in a randomised controlled trial of routine ultrasound during pregnancy. The data collected have suggested a possible link with non- right handedness and routine ultrasonography. The hypothesis was to examine any association between routine ultrasonography in utero and subsequent brain development as indicated by non-right handedness at primary school age. Although an association was found between these two parameters, the authors stress that there was no association found between routine ultrasound and impaired neurological development *(Salveson et al, 1993)*.

Two randomised controlled trials reported in 1984 *(Bakketeig et al, 1984 & Neilson et al, 1984)* looked at the possible advantages to clinical outcome of ultrasound screening in pregnancy. Both trials revealed only marginal benefits, but they did not find any evidence of deleterious effects due to ultrasound exposure. These and many other studies are reviewed in greater detail in the report of the working party published by the British Institute of Radiology 1987 *(Wells, 1987b)*.

The report made several recommendations which included the following:-

a) "Ultrasonic instruments should be designed to operate with exposure levels as low as reasonably practicable taking expense and diagnostic performance into account.

b) The search for untoward bioeffects should continue in an orderly and planned fashion.

c) Investigators who have assessed children of mothers who were exposed to ultrasound should be encouraged to undertake follow up studies."

Since these very comprehensive reviews of the literature regarding the investigations of potential hazards, further studies have shown that cavitation is unlikely to be a problem *(Evans, 1992)*.

Concern remains about the thermal dangers, particularly in respect of endprobes, for example, the vaginal probe. These have the source of ultrasound much closer to sensitive targets, in particular the early embryo *(Evans, 1992)*. Duck et al, (1990) measured the surface heat of transducers and found that probes used for Doppler techniques reached considerably higher temperatures. As the author states *"Knowledge of the extent to which the transducer is a thermal source is also necessary in the context of predictions of tissue temperature rises."*

An interesting study was undertaken by a group of two midwives, a research technologist and an obstetrician and gynaecologist in 1987. In this study, the duration of exposure time of diagnostic ultrasound was measured in 1274 women undergoing routine examination at their first visit to an ante-natal clinic. Exposure time is important because, if kept to a minimum, it will limit the amount of ultrasound energy the tissues under examination receive. Exposure is calculated by measuring the intensity of the beam, plus the time that energy is transmitted. The measured median exposure time in this study was 105 seconds *(Andrews et al, 1987)*. The authors of this study accepted that this length of time seemed short, but felt it prudent to suggest that exposure time be kept to the minimum. The relevance of the length of exposure time to issues concerning the safety of diagnostic ultrasound are discussed in this paper in the light of acoustic output levels.

As ultrasound has become established as a useful tool, operators have developed within various disciplines. These include obstetricians, radiologists, radiographers, physicists, medical practitioners, nurses and midwives. This has led to the formation of multidisciplinary societies, which includes the British Medical Ultrasound Society. This in turn is affiliated to the European Federation of Societies for Ultrasound in Medicine and Biology. The Americans have founded the American Institute of Ultrasound in Medicine.

These societies act as watch-dogs and monitor practice, including safety of the procedure. They review the literature relating to evidence of possible hazards, make recommendations and issue guide-lines. They also publish summaries of the various data and current knowledge.

2) Is the technology reliable?

Any machine is liable to break down. Any information that the machine may produce is obviously dependent on the mechanisms being maintained in good order by servicing and checking the calibration at regular and frequent intervals. It is therefore incumbent upon operators to make sure that their machinery is safe to use, and that the output levels are within the specified parameters recommended.

Another issue to be considered is: - Is the operator sufficiently trained to use the machinery? This means trained in the safe use of the technology and proficient enough to interpret the data obtained from its computer. Is the operator therefore working within the realm of 'safe practice'?

The British Medical Ultrasound Society (B.M.U.S.) has constantly addressed both these issues, but one of the biggest problems is the ease with which a recognisable picture can be obtained, lulling would be sonographers into a false sense of security regarding their own expertise.

It is a very real possibility that a mis-diagnosis of a fetal abnormality could be made by wrong interpretation causing an outcome that would be disastrous, that is, a perfectly normal fetus could be aborted, having been mistakenly diagnosed as being abnormal. Obtaining an incorrect image for the purpose of calculating gestational age or growth assessment can also cause an incorrect diagnosis to be made. Correct training meets the objective of enabling trainee sonographers to understand the physics (and therefore the potential dangers) of the machinery they are handling. It also enables them to obtain the correct image and angle of that image so that correct measuring techniques are used. Recognition of fetal abnormality is only one of the vital parts of that training.

Learning the correct technique also ensures that the operator is using the machine in a safe manner. The B.M.U.S. have issued guide-lines to aid safe practice. These include the following:-

a) There must be constant movement of the transducer over the part being scanned so that the sound waves are not being absorbed by the same tissues over any length of time.

b) Examination time should be limited to the minimum time necessary to perform an adequate diagnostic examination

c) There is no place for the trivial scan.

d) There is no place for occasional sonographers. It is recommended that a minimum weekly level of practice of one session a week should be mandatory.

e) At least one recognised course of continuing education in ultrasound should be attended every 3 years, and it is up to every sonographer to keep themselves up to date with regard to potential hazards.

Safe practice therefore means being properly trained in the technique of using the machinery, of being able to obtain a correct image and to interpret the data accurately.

In 1987, the Royal College of Obstetricians and Gynaecologists and the Royal College of Radiologists formed a joint Ultrasound Group to draw up a training programme in obstetric ultrasound for medical practitioners. They devised a training programme which included a practical as well as a theoretical component. Unfortunately it is not mandatory. Many medical practitioners still perform ultrasound examinations having had very little training in the technique *(RCOG 1987)*.

Early in 1993 a welcome agreement was reached between The British Society of Echo-cardiology, the Royal College of Midwives, College of Radiographers, Society of Vascular Technologists and the United Kingdom Association of Sonographers. It was decided that a consortium should be established to consider accreditation of sonographic courses to be called CASE *(BMUS Bulletin, May 1993)*.

Finally the doctor should consider, before using the technology of ultrasound at all, Is this the most appropriate investigation? Is this scan really necessary? Peter Wells also quoted Jennett in his presidential address: *"High technology medicine is inappropriately deployed if it is unnecessary (because the desired objective can be achieved by simpler means) unsuccessful (because the patient has a condition too advanced to respond to treatment) unsafe (because the possible complications outweigh the possible benefits) unkind (because the quality of life after rescue is not good enough, or long enough to justify the intervention) or unwise (because it diverts resources from activities that would yield greater benefits (Jennett, 1984).*

CHAPTER 3

Routine Ultrasound

Professor Iain Donald in 1974 has been reported as saying *"The day may come shortly when a routine ultrasound examination will be offered to every pregnant patient"*.

Following the concerns raised about the safety of ultrasound in the 1980s, the various watch-dog committees issued statements regarding the use of diagnostic ultrasound. The American Institute of Ultrasound in Medicine(AIUM), together with other American Associates, were very cautious and concluded with a recommendation that in their view ultrasound should not be considered as a routine screening tool in the ante-natal period *(AIUM, 1987)*.

The World Health Organisation *(1982)* recommended prudence in its use on human subjects, agreeing that the benefits outweighed presumed risks, but recommending that patients only be exposed to ultrasound for valid clinical reasons.

The Royal College of Obstetricians and Gynaecologists(RCOG, *1984)*, concluded that the safety of ultrasound was sufficiently convincing not to recommend any change in practice from the routine scanning of women between 16-18 weeks of pregnancy. Subsequently this was changed to 18 - 20 weeks gestation in order to obtain a clearer image of the fetus and therefore gain more accurate information. They also recommended, however, that large scale studies should be performed to look at the benefits of routine, as opposed to selective scanning, the latter being for clinical/medical reasons only. This has proved to be very difficult because to conduct a study of this nature comparing these two groups necessitates withholding scans from a proportion of women who might in normal circumstances receive one. Ethics committees could question the acceptability of such a study, as it might appear that one section of the population would be receiving superior treatment to the other. Studies that have been done are discussed briefly later in this chapter. The RCOG also made recommendations regarding training of operators to use the technology and that manufacturers publish the output levels after agreement of a standard level had been reached. This has subsequently been addressed. (See chapter 2).

The British Medical Ultrasound Society (1984) also issued a short statement recommending further research but agreed there was no reason to withhold ultrasound examination in the ante-natal period.

Although these statements were made in the 1980s, the content has been re-iterated at intervals, and remains valid up to the present time. The controversy regarding the use of routine screening by ultrasound in the ante-natal period still continues.

Despite the call from the various watch-dog bodies for further scientific studies to evaluate the use of ultrasound in pregnancy, very few have taken place. Bennett et al in 1982 specifically addressed the question of routine versus selective scanning in a randomised way. The results were withheld for a proportion of the subjects, but the conclusions were weakened because 30% of the concealed results were revealed to clinicians because of their "clinical anxieties". The results showed no significant difference between the two groups in terms of fetal outcome.

Eik-Nes in a letter to the Lancet in 1984 reported on a trial that had taken place in Norway during the period 1979-1980. A population of 85,000 women were divided into two groups. Half were scanned routinely, half were only scanned if there was some clinical indication. Routine ultrasound, without over-stretching hospital resources, seemed to reduce perinatal deaths, decrease morbidity levels of the infant and create a base line for the diagnosis of intra-uterine growth retardation.

Two trials performed on women in late pregnancy looked specifically at the effective use of ultrasound in the diagnosis of the growth retarded fetus (Bakketag et al, 1984 & Neilson et al, 1984). Only marginal benefits were seen in the routinely scanned group. Some other studies with relatively small sample numbers suggest that confirming the gestational age of the fetus reduces the induction rate for post maturity. There is an associated reduced incidence of babies being admitted to special care baby units because of problems associated with prematurity (Eik-Nes, 1984; Bennett et al, 1982; Bakketag et al, 1984).

The debate regarding routine scanning
Some of the arguments put forward for routine scanning include the following:-
Women deciding to participate in the maternal serum screening programme

for alpha-feto-protein levels or Downs syndrome benefit from having a scan prior to entering the programme. This is because accurate results are dependent on the gestational size of the fetus being 16-19 weeks. In one reported study, *(Brock et al, 1978)* out of a population of 21,747 women, 5.5% had a raised level of maternal serum alpha-feto-protein (MSAFP). 25% of these were found to be due to problems of fetal size or multiple gestation. An ultrasound scan performed prior to the test can thus reduce a great deal of anxiety in women recalled for further tests because of an abnormal result that is subsequently found to be due to fetal size or number. A pelvic bleed in early pregnancy can also cause a rise in the serum alpha-feto-protein levels and evidence of bleeding can be identified on the scan.

The benefits of routine scanning in early detection of multiple pregnancy has been documented by several authors from as early as 1978 *(Grennert et al, 1978; Persson et al, 1979)*. Both of these studies suggested early detection enabling subsequent careful monitoring to diagnose problems particularly growth retardation, meant that the incidence of pre-term delivery fell from 33% to 10% The perinatal morbidity rate fell from 6% to 0.6%. This rate is acknowledged to be extremely low, perhaps a more realistic rate of 8% to 1.5% is reported by MacGillivray *(1980)*. This is still high in comparison with that of singleton deliveries.

Diagnosis of a structural abnormality of the fetus can be made on a routine scan, and sometimes suspicion of chromosomal abnormalities necessitates further investigation. Women participating in a screening programme to detect, or inform them of, a risk factor for an abnormality benefit from early diagnosis.

There are also the added benefits of early diagnosis of an abnormally situated placenta. The measurements taken of the fetus at a mid trimester scan form a useful baseline on which to base patterns of growth in detecting the fetus suffering from growth related problems.

The case for routine scanning in pregnancy

One of the most controversial issues about routine scanning arises over estimation or confirmation of the gestational age of the fetus. A certain percentage of women will not be able to recall the first day of their last menstrual period (LMP) and some women have a very irregular menstrual cycle. For these an ultrasound scan is useful to estimate the expected date of confinement (EDC). It helps to prevent unnecessary and unwarranted interference when a prolonged pregnancy is suspected and acts as a baseline in monitoring the growth of the fetus.

Women who have been taking the oral contraceptive pill, which can delay ovulation, or who have experienced slight and/or irregular vaginal bleeding, may benefit from an ultrasound scan to confirm a viable pregnancy and establish the expected date of delivery. It has been estimated that these two groups form anything from 20-24% of the population of pregnant women *(Bennett et al, 1982; Warsof, 1983)*. The case for routinely scanning the proportion of women who can give the date of their last menstrual period and who have experienced no menstrual irregularities or problems in their pregnancy has been argued by several authors. Both Warsof in 1983 and Grennert in 1978 suggested that the number of women whose pregnancies exceeded 42 weeks was reduced from 12% to 6% following routine scanning. Eik-Nes (1984) came to similar conclusions. Other benefits of this study have already been mentioned.

Malcolm Pearce *(1987)* re-iterated these findings, but does not advocate changing a woman's expected date of confinement unless its prediction by ultrasound is greater, or lesser than one week in either direction.

In a more recent paper *(Giersson ,1991)* makes a very strong case for using ultrasound estimation of the expected date of confinement and ignoring the menstrual history altogether. He evaluated the use of Nagele's rule and came to the conclusion it was a very unsatisfactory method because of the inability in most instances to know precisely when ovulation took place. In his opinion most women do not have a regular menstrual cycle, there being at least two or three days departure from the mean cycle length. Women, he says, will say they have a regular cycle despite there being this albeit small deviation. "Regularity may be a relative phenomenon, that depends upon personal standards of interpretation". He argues that ultrasound gives a scientifically sound base for timing pregnancy related events which is superior to other methods. Many of course, including midwives, would argue this is an insult to women and makes pregnancy appear a potentially abnormal rather than a normal event *(Robinson & Beech, 1993; Flint 1987)*.

In 1992 Luck reported on a prospective study he had undertaken over the four year period 1988-1991 inclusive. All pregnant women attending the hospital during this time were offered scans at 19 weeks gestation. 96% of the total accepted. 140 fetal abnormalities were diagnosed, enabling termination of pregnancy to be offered for lethal malformations, preparation for delivery for others and parents were prepared for the outcome. Benefits included a reduced number of post-natal investigations for the baby. The author claimed a tremendous financial saving, far outweighing running costs.

Beverley Beech (Maternity Rights Campaigner, 1987) estimated that the Department of Health are spending £15,000,000 a year on scanning women in pregnancy. She based this assumption on the cost of a scan being £14. Costing a scan, however, can be difficult. Running costs vary according to who operates the machine, and who interprets the results, (with regard to the salaries involved) the type of the machine, the time it takes to perform each examination, the types of recording equipment used, the reporting methods and the number of scans performed during each session. It could be argued that having purchased the machinery, the more it is used, the cheaper the individual scans become. It is difficult to assess the amount of electricity used in running a scanning department, especially as work load might vary from day to day according to how much the machine is in use. Costing is something that can be used on either side of the debate. Advocates supporting routine scanning could argue that screening reduces costs of supporting numbers of handicapped children. They would also argue that these numbers are reduced, not only because most parents accept termination for the fetus shown to be lethally malformed, but also that careful monitoring of the fetus reduces the numbers compromised by intra-uterine growth retardation. It also enables those fetuses with potentially life threatening conditions to receive the best treatment, at the best possible location, at the earliest possible time, thus reducing the level of any handicap. This is because adequate preparations can be made before the child is born

The psychological benefits women receive from having an early scan are documented by Campbell *(1982)*, having studied two groups of women having scans. One group could see the screen, the images being deciphered for them by the operator. The other group looked into the back of the monitor and could see nothing, but were told that everything appeared to be all right. A questionnaire given to the two groups revealed that the group able to see the fetus moving about on the screen had a more positive attitude to their pregnancy and stronger emotional ties to the baby than the other group. Other studies done by Reading *(Reading & Cox, 1982 & 1988; Reading & Platt, 1985)* confirm these findings, and suggest that maternal anxieties are reduced after having seen the moving fetus for themselves.

The case against routine scanning in pregnancy

The arguments for routine scanning have been very forceful during the past decade but professionals are beginning to realise that, although scanning might reduce some problems, it can produce some of its own. Adrian Grant is reported (in the Nursing Times *1987)* as having raised the issue that it might also raise new dilemmas for parents. When minor abnormalities are identified, they give cause to great anxiety until the baby is born, as the meaning of these minor aberrations is very often still unknown. Scans in this instance are more anxiety provoking than helpful.

Josephine Green in her study examining the psychological effects of fetal diagnosis on pregnant women , discovered that whereas ultrasound scanning is favourably viewed where it happens, where it is not used routinely women do not feel deprived. Both groups felt that the ante-natal care they received was the best *(Green, 1990)*.

Her conclusions about the psychological aspects were that many of the studies reporting a bonding with the fetus were over emphasised. Much depended on the quality of the communication with the operator and the level of anxiety experienced prior to the procedure.

A report from the reporters of 'Which' discussing the place of routine scanning, recommended that if routine scanning were to be offered to women it should be stressed that it is **NOT** an essential part of their ante-natal care *(WHICH, 1985)*.

Further doubt has been placed on the effectiveness of routine scanning by a meta analysis of four randomised controlled trials evaluating the effect of various outcome measures *(Bucher et al, 1993)*. The question asked was "Does routine ultrasound scanning in pregnancy improve outcome in pregnancy? Perinatal mortality, rate of miscarriages, number of live births, Apgar scores, and numbers of inductions were examined. In all 15,935 pregnancies were included in the study, 7,992 of which had a routine scan and 7,943 were used as a control group and were scanned if there was a clinical reason only.

There was no difference in the live birth rate between the two groups. Perinatal mortality was lower in the routinely scanned group, due in the main to induced abortion for fetal abnormalities that was reported in one of the trials. There was no significant difference in perinatal morbidity between the two groups as measured by an Apgar score of less than 7 at 1 minute. The authors came to the conclusion there were no real benefits to routine scanning in pregnancy.

Tennerman et al, *(1991)* came to a similar conclusion for scanning in the first trimester.

Writing in 'Professional Nurse' in July, 1990, Joanne Whelton states "*Whether or not we agree with screening, midwives have a duty to provide clients with up to date information regarding the tests available"* The midwives responsibility is stated clearly in the Midwife's Code of Practice *"to prescribe or advise on the examinations necessary for the earliest possible diagnosis of pregnancies at risk." (UKCC, 1991)*

Probably the most important point is that women are given a choice. Many women are persuaded by anxious clinicians to have a scan for some apparently good clinical reason, without being told of its potential to detect fetal abnormalities. Many view the experience as a chance to have a preview of a baby they will have in their arms at some future date, and bring partners and family to share in what they see as an exciting experience. To have informed choice it is imperative they are given all the relevant information prior to accepting the offer of a scan. This applies whether it is part of a routine screening programme, or a selective scan offered because of a suspicion of a medical or obstetric problem.

CHAPTER 4

Ethical Considerations

In 1992 at a symposium on the Issues in Fetal Medicine, Mr. S. Walkinshaw of Liverpool Maternity Hospital said that in his opinion the ethical issues surrounding pre-natal screening by ultrasound had never been properly addressed. He stressed the need for counselling for every parent and suggested that no pre-natal screening programme should be introduced until a counsellor had been appointed.

In 1991 Chervenak and McCullough addressing the morality of scanning women in an article called *"Ethics: an emerging sub-discipline of obstetric ultrasound,"* wrote*" Ethics is an emerging subdiscipline of obstetric ultrasound because there are clinical dimensions of obstetric ultrasound that only ethics can identify and address."*

In pursuing the best interests of the client, it is not just the clinicians perspective of the best interests that need to be taken into consideration. The client may have a different set of values, beliefs and perhaps other related interests to take into consideration, as well as the advice of a well meaning clinician.

This respect for the clients' autonomy is re-iterated in the Patients' Charter. The woman has a choice. To make a choice she needs to be informed. This whole ethical principle is captured in the principle of informed consent.

Richard Wells *(1986)* discussing informed consent in the Nursing Times, makes the observation that very often nurses and midwives, although concerned that clients are fully informed about all aspects of care, if acting in a subservient role to some consultants may be guilty of withholding relevant information. He also suggests that emotional feelings might prevent a midwife from being able to express a rational informed opinion.

To be a good advocate for the womant, therefore, the midwife mus have sufficient knowledge about the technology and exactly what it is likely to reveal. She must also have the emotional equilibrium to be able to remain unbiased when inviting the woman to partake of the screening so that the woman herself can truly make an informed choice.

Ultrasound screening is now available to most women and the invitation to participate is likely in itself to raise anxiety levels *(Marteau, 1990)*. Sometimes even if the scan reveals no obvious abnormality, anxiety levels will remain raised until the baby is born, just because the thought of possible malformation has been put into the woman's mind by offering the test.

Marteau(1990) suggests that anxiety levels can be reduced by preparation, either in the form of a written explanation, or by discussing the procedure during the course of a consultation. As has already been stated, the RCOG advise written explanation (Chapter 2). Written explanation should not preclude the opportunity for discussion. Both would be ideal.

During preparation, several issues need to be addressed - Why the test is available; why the scan is being offered; and why it is thought to be a good thing. As has already been stated in Chapter 3, many women do not see scanning as a screening test, but it is looked upon as the highlight of their pregnancy. It is important that the women are informed that it can pick up certain abnormalities and are not told that it is to "make sure the baby is all right". There are many conditions of the fetus that cannot be detected by ultrasound. The type of abnormalities that can be picked up, or suspected, should be described. Making sure the baby is alright implies that if it is not alright, the condition can be rectified. This was discussed by Josephine Green in her study (*1991*). Ultrasound can still only detect a relatively small number of abnormalities, even if this is the specific reason for performing the scan.Women have come to expect the perfect baby. Screening has come to be seen as the means of detecting the "not so perfect baby".

It must also be explained exactly what the test involves and when the results will be available. Parents also need to know if the scan operator will tell them the results, or if the results will be sent to the clinician.

Other issues worry women and need to be discussed. For instance, in the likelihood of any abnormalities being discovered, what are the likely outcomes available to them? Very often the only option that is seemingly available is termination of the pregnancy, but is that the only option? It is implicit in most screening programmes that there should be a reduction in the birth of babies with congenital abnormalities which are diagnosed in pregnancy, and the only way to achieve this is by termination of pregnancy. The fact that some abnormalities, if treated immediately, can mean the child has every chance of leading a perfectly normal life, (provided that a suitable place for delivery is arranged), needs to be explained. There are many conditions of the fetus that are amenable to intra-uterine and/or neonatal treatment. There are other conditions that might have a better prognosis if the fetus were to have an instrumental, rather than a normal vaginal delivery. A scan will alert the professional team of certain abnormalities, or suspicion of an abnormality, so that the best possible care can be given for each individual woman and her family.

If the scan is thought to be advisable to monitor fetal growth, just as much explanation is needed, but it is rarely given. Casual remarks that the fetus might be small can cause tremendous anxiety, and women sent for ultrasound investigation for this reason often wait a week or more before they can discuss the results with a midwife or obstetrician.

According to Marteau(1990) *"Staff training is the cornerstone of a successful screening programme, yet this is one of the more neglected aspects of running screening programmes."* Many staff, she says, think they know how to counsel women, but they very seldom have the necessary skills. They do need training. *"Counselling is the process through which one person helps another by purposeful conversation in an understanding manner" (Jones, 1978).* In relation to making an informed choice about whether to participate in a screening programme, including ultrasound, counselling can help parents clarify their situation and face the decision with less anxiety. The purpose of counselling is to assist them to make their own decision from the choices available. This choice should be voluntary, there should be no coercion. Once the parents have decided, their choice should be respected. Very often pressure is brought to bear upon women to change their minds as the pregnancy progresses. Various reasons are given to influence them, sometimes spurious and amounting to a form of emotional blackmail. Health care providers should be there to give parents support in whatever they decide to do.

Ultrasound policies and protocols

Because of the issues discussed in previous chapters regarding safety, the concentration needed to perform scans effectively, thereby gaining the maximum amount of information in the minimum amount of time, and taking into consideration the ethical issues, it is usually necessary to form a set of policies within ultrasound departments. Thought needs to be given to the consequences of having visitors allowed in to see the scan. Children running around distract some sonographers, disturb their concentration and thus lengthen the time of the scan. Information given during the procedure might be restricted if friends or neighbours are present, rather than next of kin. Health professionals are also sharply divided on the question of whether the sex of the fetus should be divulged to the parents.

Good communication with the obstetrician is essential so that problems can be discussed immediately, and trust between members of the professional team is a prime requisite.

Practical Preparations

Having decided to have a scan the physical preparation depends largely upon the period of gestation and the reason for the scan. In the first trimester of pregnancy the maternal urinary bladder needs to be full. This is because the uterus and its contents are pushed up out of the pelvis when the bladder is full and can be viewed abdominally.

When scanning to localise a placenta, the internal cervical os needs to be visible so that its relationship to the lower edge of the placenta can be ascertained. Again, the maternal urinary bladder needs to be full in order that a clear view abdominally can be obtained. It is not usually necessary for the woman to change into a gown for an ultrasound scan these days as the gel which is now used does not ruin or harm clothes like the oils which were formerly used. The gel is easily wiped off after the scan has been completed.

It should be noted that scanning the obese woman can present difficulties. They manifest themselves mainly in two ways:-
a) the distance between the transducer and the fetus is greater and the soundwaves are therefore weaker
b) the fat tissue absorbs the soundwaves making the image less distinct.

On completion of the scan women need to be told the results, or when they are likely to receive the results, and given the opportunity to ask any questions.

CHAPTER 5

Measurements used in Ultrasound

Some of the earliest uses of ultrasound in obstetrics were concerned with the estimation or confirmation of the gestational age of the pregnancy, and monitoring fetal growth. As the resolution of the machines improved it became possible to examine the fetus for abnormalities. All these investigations require various uses of measurements. Some of the basic measurements used will be described in this chapter, together with their uses and limitations.

Linear Measurements
Crown Rump Length

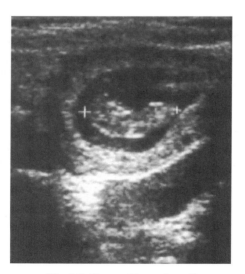

Fig. 5.1 Crown Rump Length

This is a linear measurement taken from the crown of the head to the rump. The attitude of the fetus or embryo,that is the degree of flexion or extension, does have a bearing on the accuracy of the measurement. The ideal is to freeze the image when the embryo is stretched and the longest axis is then measured. Flexion becomes more marked as gestational age increases. To measure the crown rump length, it is obviously necessary to visualise the entire embryo, so this measurement cannot be used once the image gets too big to be seen on the screen in the correct perspective. It is therefore usually used in the first trimester of pregnancy only.

It is quite difficult to obtain an accurate measurement on small images that move at a fast rate and are very often curled up. It is also difficult to examine them for fetal anomalies because they are so small that only the most major defects are visible. When the correct image is obtained it does give one of the most precise assessments of gestational age. There are considerable differences between the measurements over a period of just one week because the embryo grows at such a rapid rate. The range of measurements equivalent to gestational age is narrow, the two standard deviations above and below the mean being equivalent to only a day or two.

Some of the difficulties associated with scanning in the first trimester have been overcome with the advent of the vaginal probe. Very accurate measurements of the embryo can be obtained, but it is not always such an acceptable form of scanning as the abdominal route so, unless there is a compelling reason for its use in the first trimester, it is not the usual method.

Although Robinson and Fleming*(1975)* advocated estimating the gestational age of the fetus in the first trimester by use of the crown rump length, it was superseded by the bi-parietal diameter as the most useful measurement for the purpose.

Studies performed at King's College Hospital in the early 1980s suggested that because of the difficulties experienced in scanning the embryo, it was wiser to delay scanning until other measurements could more easily be obtained *(Warsof, 1983)*. These measurements were more likely to be accurate and reproducible. The scan could also be performed at a time when women were attending the hospital for other screening tests, thus limiting the number of clinic attendances.

The Bi-Parietal Diameter (BPD)

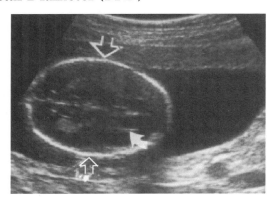

Fig. 5.2 Open arrows indicate parietal eminences - solid arrow indicates ventricular horn

This is the longitudinal measurement between the parietal eminences and is the maximum transverse diameter of the fetal skull. Again the correct image must be obtained and frozen and the callipers placed between them. This measurement is useful for estimation of gestational age from 12 weeks to approximately 24-28 weeks. It can, of course, be taken until term, but head shapes can influence its accuracy in the third trimester and the range or spread of a particular measurement to gestational age becomes so wide that, after 28 weeks, it is impossible to use it for accurate estimation of gestational age.

It does have a use in the third trimester since, in combination with other measurements, it can be used to monitor fetal growth. Other measurements, however, can give a more accurate picture of the state of the fetus with regard to growth and fetal well being.

Femur Length (FL)

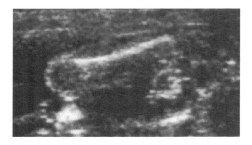

Fig. 5.3 Femur Length

This is the longitudinal measurement along the long axis of the femur. It is useful in assessing the gestational age of the fetus in the second trimester but, like the other measurements, the range equal to gestational age becomes so broad that, after 28 weeks, it cannot be used for that purpose. It can be a useful parameter, in conjunction with others, for monitoring fetal growth and in the detection of fetal abnormalities.

When assessing the gestational age of the fetus in the second trimester it is useful to combine more than one measurement, usually the bi-parietal diameter and the femur length, or the bi-parietal diameter and the crown rump length. A more accurate estimation of the expected date of delivery can be obtained by the use of more than one parameter. If correlation of the two is not possible a fetal anomaly of some kind should be suspected.

Other measurements can be used to estimate gestational age, or can be used in combination with those already mentioned. These include intra-orbital measurements, or the diameter of the cerebellum.

NON LINEAR MEASUREMENTS

Head Circumference (HC)

This can be measured at the same time as the bi-parietal diameter. The same image is required. It is obtained by tracing round the perimeter of the fetal skull and can be used in the assessment of gestational age up until 28 weeks. The head circumference is usually used in combination with other measurements to monitor fetal growth. Most sonographers find it useful to measure it at the same time as the bi-parietal diameter so that a baseline is available for future reference, should it become necessary.

Abdominal Circumference (AC)

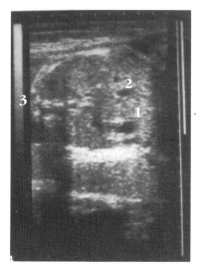

Having obtained the correct image, which is a cross section of the fetal abdomen (showing a short section of the (1) stomach, (2) umbilical vein, fetal liver, and (3) a cross section of the spine), a trace of the perimeter is obtained. This is a very useful measurement to use when assessing fetal growth because of fat deposition in the fetal liver. This is reduced in the growth retarded fetus and increased in macrosomia.

A useful method of monitoring fetal growth is measuring both the head circumference and the abdominal circumference. The ratio head circumference/abdominal circumference helps to distinguish between two types of growth retardation. Asymmetrical growth retardation is characterised by a diminishing abdominal circumference but the head circumference remains within normal limits. This is sometimes referred to as !brain sparing , that is the brain continues to receive sufficient nutrients and continues to develop, whereas the fat and glycogen deposits in the liver become depleted as the fetus is compromised.

In symmetrical growth retardation, the fetus suffers from insufficient nutrition which affects both the brain and other organs. The head circumference as well as the abdominal circumference are reduced. This more serious condition is very often associated with chromosomal abnormalities.

It is very often difficult to differentiate between the growth retarded fetus and the small for dates fetus. The latter is small from the very first scan in the first trimester of pregnancy. The cause is often attributed to incorrect dates and the woman is therefore given a revised expected date of delivery. More often than not it is caused by a genetic disorder.

Volume Measurements

Gestational sac volumes are sometimes useful in the first trimester to distinguish between the ≅blighted ovum and an early gestational sac. Various operators have tried to measure the volume of liquor later in pregnancy with little success. Amounts of liquor in the third trimester are often commented on subjectively by the sonographer, especially polyhydramnios and oligohydramnios. Sometimes pools of liquor, once identified on scan, are measured by linear measurements to give an indication of their depth and this gives an indication of relative amounts.

Fetal Weight

Formulae have been developed to give an estimate of fetal weight. They include various parameters that are used in combination. These various combinations give reasonable accuracy. The one that is the most accurate is a combination of the abdominal circumference and the femur length *(Hadlock et al, 1985)*.

It is quite useful to estimate fetal weight in cases of pre-term labour, breech presentation, diabetes or previous lower segment caesarean section, when anticipating vaginal delivery.

Collecting and charting the data

The British Medical Ultrasound Society has, after a series of workshops, recommended the data and charts that should be used when examining and measuring the fetus. They have come to these conclusions after searching all papers concerned with ultrasonic fetal measurement, of which there are many. It is therefore hoped that in the future there will be greater uniformity in the practice of making routine ultrasound measurements.

Estimation of Gestational Age by Ultrasound

One of the most controversial issues associated with ultrasound in the ante-natal period is estimation of gestational age.

Women who are certain of the date of the first day of their last menstrual period, have a regular menstrual cycle with no underlying medical or obstetric problems, and who have not recently been taking the oral contraceptive pill do not necessarily require a scan for estimation of gestational age. (see Chapter 3) It is an issue that causes women great distress, especially those who know when they conceived. Very often the problem is not one of fetal measurement, but how that measurement is reported and subsequently interpreted and/or applied to the clinical situation.

On occasions a woman who has had several scans during her pregnancy may have her expected date of delivery (EDD) altered on each and every occasion. This might be because the sonographer has reported the measurements of the fetus in terms of equating them to a certain gestational age. The following example might help to clarify this phenomenon.

A woman might have a scan at 16 weeks which confirms that the measurements taken at that time are within normal limits for that gestation. At a subsequent ante-natal clinic visit at 32 weeks gestation it is thought that the fetus is small for that gestational age and a scan is requested. The report then states that the fetal measurements equate with a fetus of 30 weeks gestation. Incorrect interpretation of these results might result in altering the expected date of confinement. The real problem is that this 32 week fetus has not grown at the normal rate, it has only reached the size of a normal 30 week fetus. A diagnosis of growth retardation therefore might be more appropriate.

Many sonographers have limited obstetric knowledge so that correlation of the results to the clinical situation are left to the clinicians. In a large imaging department the scan on any particular woman is performed in isolation, being unrelated to previous scans or the woman's obstetric history.

There are two approaches, to the so called 'dating scan'. The gestational age is estimated because the woman has no idea of the date of the first day of her last menstrual period, or has a history of irregular menstrual cycles, has recently taken the oral contraceptive pill, or has simply failed to keep a record of her menstrual cycles. Fetal measurements are taken and correlated to the mean for a particular gestational age. The expected date of delivery is estimated from that point.

The other approach is designed to confirm gestational age of the fetus. In this instance the expected date of delivery is known having been calculated by the midwife or doctor, usually using Naegele's rule. Measurements of the fetus are taken and compared with the normal range of measurements equivalent to the known gestational age.

Conflict arises when there is an apparent discrepancy. Reasons for this can lie with both the operator/interpreter and/or the woman; discussion can usually resolve any problems. An agreed expected date of delivery is then given. Problems of interpretation can arise when the sonographer fails to take into account the range of measurements for any given gestational age. The two standard deviations above and below the mean are very often disregarded. There are also instances, although rare, where the measurements can fall outside these parameters. If the woman is confident that her dates are correct, it is inappropriate to alter her expected date of delivery. The fetus might very well be small or large for dates. Genetic abnormality should be suspected if it is very small.

Very few women have a regular 28 day menstrual cycle. Often when women are asked if they commence their menstrual period on the same day every month they have to admit that they have either a shorter or a longer cycle. Some have very irregular cycles, several days less or more than 28 days, and the cycle changes each month. Many have been taking the oral contraceptive pill which very often delays ovulation. Some women calculate their expected date of delivery from the last day of their menstrual period.

Altering the expected date of delivery when the woman is not in agreement should therefore be a rare occurrence. In fact altering it at all is questionable unless there is more than 10-14 days discrepancy with the previously given date, whether it was calculated from the last menstrual period or from a previous scan.

If communication with women about their scans were given more of a priority, much distress caused by worry over dates and the size of the baby would be avoided.

CHAPTER 6

The Place of Scanning in the First Trimester of Pregnancy

Ultrasound scanning in early pregnancy can be very useful. Women may experience problems such as bleeding per vaginam or abdominal pain. These possible complications can cause a lot of anxiety at a time when the woman might be feeling very miserable and suffering a variety of unpleasant symptoms. Until ultrasound became so readily available many problems remained unsolved until they either disappeared, resolved, or became so acute that they developed into an obstetric emergency.

The advent of the vaginal probe in the first trimester has made visualisation easier because the structures of the pelvis and its contents, including the tiny embryo, are much closer to the probe. This enables the structures to be seen in much greater detail.

In particular, the vaginal probe has revolutionised the diagnosis and treatment of ectopic pregnancy. The tubes can be seen and examined directly for any distension. In practice the fallopian tubes are often hidden by loops of bowel and are often very difficult to visualise. However they can often be seen if:-
a) Fluid is present around the adnexa e.g. following ovulation or tubal rupture.
b) Abnormal pathology is present e.g. hydrosalpinx, pyosalpinx.
c) The presence of an ectopic pregnancy may be revealed as an echogenic mass lying between the uterus and ovary; often referred to as a "polo-sign".

In a study performed in Finland in 1990 to test the efficacy of vaginal scanning for this purpose, two hundred women with symptoms of bleeding plus abdominal pain were scanned. Direct diagnosis was possible using the vaginal route for scanning in 93% of the group *(Carriatore et al, 1990)*. Writing in the British Medical Journal in 1992 Goswamy states, *"The use of transvaginal scanning in early detection and treatment of ectopic pregnancy may ultimately have a greater impact on maternal mortality than any other recent development in gynaecology."* When using the vaginal probe there is no need for the woman to have a full bladder. The sonographer can differentiate between ovarian and tubal masses and a technique of injecting directly into the fetal sac in cases of ectopic pregnancy, resulting in spontaneous reabsorption of the fetus can be used, thus obviating the need of further surgery *(Goswamy, 1992).*

Diagnosis of ectopic pregnancy by using abdominal scanning is difficult. A positive diagnosis is usually made on the absence of a fetal sac within the uterine cavity, together with an adenexal mass and/or the presence of free fluid in the pelvis. Human chorionic gonadotrophin (HCG) levels in the maternal serum are usually assessed to confirm a pregnancy. A fetal sac outside the uterus is rarely seen.

Transvaginal scanning makes it a lot easier to visualise the early embryo, especially in obese women, or women with a retroverted uterus. Abdominal scanning can be very difficult in these instances because the beam from the transducer needs to reach considerable depths for an image to be seen. Ultrasound energy is lost in the surrounding tissues which results in very poor images. This necessitates filling the maternal bladder to extraordinary proportions to create an acoustic window, making the woman extremely uncomfortable.This is very unpleasant for her at a time when nausea and vomiting are likely symptoms and frequency of micturition, which is also a common disorder of early pregnancy, sometimes makes this impossible. Vaginal scanning therefore becomes the route of choice.

When detailed examination of the early embryo is required, scanning by introducing the probe into the vagina enables the sonographer to examine the development of the embryo from close quarters. The embryological structures are observed one week earlier than with abdominal scanning. This can be advantageous when problems arise with the pregnancy, or when a diagnosis of a suspected anomaly is required at this stage. A scan using the vaginal probe is particularly useful when a family history necessitates early screening of a possible genetic disorder.

Vaginal scanning is usually accepted by women, particularly when they are anxious because of uncertainties about their pregnancy. However in scanning departments where it is undertaken, clear policy guide-lines need to be established regarding its use. Indiscriminate use, it has been suggested, could be construed as a form of rape. Abdominal scanning is more user friendly and is still the preferred route, provided the required information can be obtained.

Circumstances in which ultrasound scanning can be useful, in the first trimester of pregnancy are listed below:-

1) At the commencement of a screening programme for the diagnosis of fetal anomalies, or prior to investigations for genetic disorders, for example prior to chorionic villus sampling or maternal serum screening.

2) To monitor fetal growth and well being by establishing a baseline on which to assess the results and to eliminate the possibility of any complications such as fibroids, and to detect a multiple pregnancy.

3) To investigate the cause of vaginal bleeding.

4) To investigate the cause of excessive vomiting in pregnancy which could be associated with multiple pregnancy or hydatidiform mole.

5) To investigate the cause of abdominal pain.

6) To unravel the mystery of ambiguous pregnancy testing results.

7) To monitor the pregnancy following treatment for infertility.

8) As part of a routine scanning programme to confirm or establish gestational age.

The ultrasound picture in early pregnancy

The fetal sac can be identified as early as five weeks gestation and the pulsating embryo from six weeks, thus establishing viability. The embryo can be measured from end to end along the crown rump length to establish or confirm gestational age. (see Chapter 5) The presence of any ovarian or uterine masses can be detected. Any gross abnormality of the embryo can be identified from approximately ten weeks gestation, for example, anencephaly, thereby negating the need for any further investigation, because the abnormality is identified and diagnosed immediately. By nine weeks the head can be distinguished from the body. Total body movements and a fetal heart can be identified. Usually the yolk sac is seen.

By twelve weeks the limb buds can be identified - when using the vaginal probe they can be seen at 8-8.5 weeks gestation.

The presence of a yolk sac within the fetal sac is thought by some to be a good prognostic sign in the case of threatened abortion. Its absence can mean a poor prognosis.

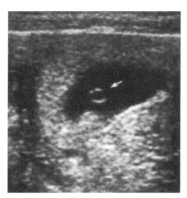

*Fig. 6.1 Fetal sac magnified
arrow indicates yolk sac*

The use of scanning prior to entering a screening programme has already been discussed. Chorionic villus sampling, (the technique of removing some of the placental tissue so that a karyotype of the cells can be performed, to screen for those at risk of some genetic disorder), is usually undertaken at approximately 10 weeks gestation. It can, in theory, be undertaken at any stage of the pregnancy, but the advantage of an early test is that if termination is offered for a positive result it can be performed during the first trimester.

Vaginal Bleeding

One of the most common problems in early pregnancy, causing a great deal of anxiety to many women, is vaginal bleeding. Ultrasound can very often expedite a diagnosis and thus save some of the anxieties.

Women with heavy vaginal bleeding , accompanied by pain and the passage of blood clots, are likely to have evidence of a dilating cervix. In these instances abortion is inevitable and there is no reason to perform a scan. Evacuation of the uterus is the best course of action if vaginal bleeding remains heavy, as the abortion is probably incomplete. When an abortion is thought to be incomplete an ultrasound scan can detect the presence of retained products of conception. If no retained products are detected, the examination saves the woman undergoing an unnecessary anaesthetic and dilatation of the cervix and curretage of the uterus.

Bleeding in early pregnancy without pain and cervical dilatation can cause intense anxiety for the woman and some degree of a dilemma for the clinicians. Ambiguous pregnancy test results, at this stage,can often add to the confusion. Repeated pregnancy testing can be an added source of anxiety as consistent positive results may not always corroborate the clinical picture. Hormonal levels can remain high for some time following the death of the embryo, as is seen in the case of a missed abortion. Viability can be determined by performing a scan. Again, if there is doubt, the crown rump length can be measured and repeated after a few days. If the measurement has not increased and there is no movement or sign of fetal pulsation, a diagnosis of missed abortion is confirmed.

Sometimes the fertilised ovum is blighted causing the development to be inhibited. A large fetal sac is seen with few, if any, echoes within it. This is sometimes referred to as an anembryonic,or anoeploid pregnancy. Very often women suffering from missed abortion or an anembryonic pregnancy recount histories of 'no longer feeling pregnant', but find it hard to accept because they have not experienced the outward signs of a miscarriage. Sometimes the images on the screen, shown with sensitivity, will help them come to terms with the diagnosis. For some women this will give them time to adjust to the loss. *"It is extremely difficult for a mother to disassociate herself from her unborn baby, to accept that although she herself lives, the baby within her does not". (Jolly, 1989a)*

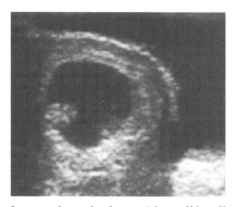

Fig. 6.2 Blighted ovum - large fetal sac with small bundle of fetal echoes

On a happier note many women, having experienced bleeding in early pregnancy, can be reassured by having a scan and seeing a live fetus moving about on the screen. Viability thus demonstrated can, of course, be confirmed at the time of the scan only. There is some evidence to suggest that showing a woman a live fetus on the screen can do much to relax her and improve the prognosis in cases of threatened abortion. Women suffering from habitual abortion should, some authorities advocate, be scanned at regular intervals so that the relaxed state can be assured, thus improving prognosis. The value of this repeated examination of the embryo has not been proved. It must be assessed against the unknown, potential hazard of repeated doses of ultrasound energy on the developing embryo.

The Vanishing Twin Phenomenon

Very often vaginal bleeding in early pregnancy is thought to be the loss of one embryo in a twin pregnancy. This is sometimes termed 'the vanishing twin'. It is diagnosed when the ultrasound scan reveals an image of two sacs, one of which is empty. The appearance of two sacs often happens following a bleed from the placental site. It may be caused by separation of the chorionic membrane from the uterine wall which gives a very similar appearance on ultrasound to an empty fetal sac. Diagnosis of the 'lost twin' can easily be confused with sub-chorionic haemorrhage.

Loss of a twin in utero causes great distress to women *"The reality is that often the distress and bereavement felt for the dead baby totally outweighs the fact that there is a living child" (Jolly, 1989b)*. Diagnosis of a multiple pregnancy should only be made, therefore, when an embryo is identified within each sac, and loss of a twin only when a multiple pregnancy has been diagnosed on a previous occasion. Approximately half of the women who are suspected of having a twin pregnancy by ultrasound in the first trimester will eventually deliver twins, a further third will deliver a singleton, the remainder miscarry *(Robinson & Caines, 1977; Varma, 1979)*.

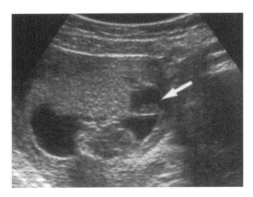

Fig. 6.3 Arrow indicates embryo no longer viable

Excessive vomiting in the first trimester

This is a particularly distressing problem. Ultrasound can sometimes aid the discovery of the cause. Very high levels of human chorionic gonadotrophin in the urine or maternal serum, accompanied by a vaginal loss which is described as being 'bitty' and brownish in colour, suggests trophoblastic disease in the form of a hydatidiform mole. This has a very characteristic appearance on ultrasound. The placenta appears big with large oedematous villi and the ovaries often contain theca lutein cysts. The woman feels ill with the accompanying abdominal discomfort and nausea and/or vomiting due to the high HCG and oestrogen levels. Ultrasound can not only aid in the diagnosis of this condition but also be used to monitor the ovaries as they return to normal following evacuation of the mole. The reduction in size and eventual disappearance of the cysts can be observed.

Excessive vomiting very often occurs in cases of multiple pregnancy, again due to the high hormonal levels produced from the increased trophoblastic activity.

Where no obvious cause for excessive vomiting is found the woman can, to a large extent, be reassured which might in itself help to ease her symptoms.

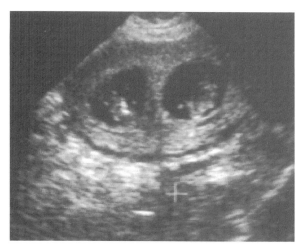

Fig. 6.4 Twins

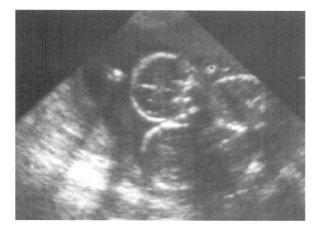

Fig. 6.5 Triplets

Monitoring follicular development and confirming the pregnancy of women having treatment for infertility

Follicles can be seen as echo free areas in the ovary and they can be measured. A developing follicle can be monitored by ultrasound as it grows to approximately 18-30 millimetres, and ovulation can be diagnosed by its subsequent collapse. This is done by examining the woman on alternate days.

If the ovaries are stimulated by Clomiphene or Perganol, multiple follicles may be seen to develop. Follicles measuring over 8 millimeters are measured at each visit. When the optimum size is reached by two or three follicles and no more in Perganol stimulated cycles, the woman receives an injection of human chorionic gonadotrophin. For women who wish to proceed to in vitro fertilization the ova are retrieved from the ruptured follicles, fertilised and returned to the uterus. The uterus is then scanned after a short interval to ensure that a pregnancy has been established and to count the number of sacs, or embryos, that have successfully implanted.

Routine Scanning

Routine scanning in the first trimester can reveal many of the problems described in this chapter. A study done by Tennerman in Belgium in 1991 found 25 women out of a group of 1011 had abnormalities. Expected or not, the results of an abnormality are devastating for the woman. Her distress can be exacerbated if it takes place during a hospital visit when she knows that other women are enjoying the experience of seeing their normal baby on the screen for the first time.

Excitement and overwhelming maternal feelings are very common during the scan. Many women are delighted to see the moving fetus on the screen and say they feel pregnant for the first time. Concealing abnormal findings from the woman, or delaying discussion of adverse findings, or indeed a diagnosis, by referring reports to clinicians who see them at a future date is unkind. Clinicians should be available to discuss adverse findings immediately they are discovered if operators are unable to divulge the information themselves. It is impossible to mislead a woman if a live healthy fetus cannot be demonstrated on the screen.

When a woman agrees to accept routine scanning it may well be that her first scan will take place in the first trimester of pregnancy. For the majority of women it will take place in the second trimester which will be the subject of the next chapter.

CHAPTER 7

Scanning in the Second Trimester of Pregnancy

Following the deliberations of the working party of the Royal College of Obstetricians and Gynaecologists in 1984, a recommendation was made that the then common practice of offering a routine ultrasound examination to women between 16-18 weeks of pregnancy should continue *(RCOG 1984)*. This reiterated Stuart Campbell's recommendation of the year before, when writing in Recent Advances in Clinics in Obstetrics and Gynaecology *(Campbell & Pearce, 1983)*. He predicted that, in the near future, every fetus would have the opportunity of having an anatomical scan at 18 weeks gestation.

The sequence and the format of that scan, recommended at that time, remains the basis of the examination today. The only difference is that the resolution of the machinery has improved so that an even more detailed examination is possible. Not only can structural defects of the fetus be recognised, but minute deviations from the normal can be identified leading the operator to look for patterns of abnormalities that might suggest chromosomal defects. These minor defects are often alluded to as 'chromosome markers.' Very often chromosomal defects are identified in the neonate by identification of a syndrome. The syndrome comprising of a series of minor anomalies that lead to a suspicion of an abnormal chromosomal complement. This will result in a series of tests which will either confirm or deny that suspicion. If a chromosome marker is observed on ultrasound, the sonographer is alerted to look for other markers that might add up to the diagnosis of a syndrome. Further investigations, for example, amniocentesis, can then be carried out to enable fetal cells to be karyotyped for examination of the fetal chromosome complement. Some genetic abnormalities can also be identified in a similar way.

There are to date several hundred conditions which may be visualised antenatally by ultrasound, but some are so rare that they will not be seen in the ordinary unit. Large referral units only become expert in their detection.

The arguments for and against routine scanning in the ante-natal period have already been discussed, but whether every woman should have such a detailed examination. as suggested above, is an additional issue and is also debatable. A lot will depend upon the machinery, the amount of time allowed for the examination and the expertise of the sonographer.

It has already been argued that women accepting a scan should be aware that abnormalities of the fetus can be discovered on any routine scan, even if the primary request for a scan was for a reason other than that of looking for abnormalities of the fetus. Detailed examination to exclude abnormalities suggests to the woman and her family that the baby she will have in her arms at term will be absolutely perfect. This is particularly so if the offer of screening for abnormalities is 'sold' to women by telling them ultrasound is offered *'to make sure your baby is all right'*. Women have come to expect a perfect baby, but even if the baby when born appears perfectly normal it might not fulfil that woman's perception of her perfect baby. The concept of the perfect baby, because a scan has eliminated the possibility of any abnormality, is a dangerous one to convey. Sometimes minor abnormalities can be missed. Subsequent events in the pregnancy or at delivery might also result in a less than 'perfect' baby. So even if the scan reveals no obvious abnormalities it is unwise to say that the baby will be perfectly normal at birth. Womens' expectations may still not be fulfilled. The sonographer must be very careful, therefore, when scanning for abnormalities of the fetus about communicating the results to the woman and her family, even if everything appears to be normal at the time of the scan. Minor anomalies can be discovered on scan which might or might not have any clinical significance. Any such discovery can cause intense anxiety until the baby is born, when either further investigations can be carried out, or the true picture is instantly seen.

Dr Margaret McNay, Consultant Obstetrician Sonographer, writing in the British Medical Ultrasound Bulletin in 1991 said, *"ultrasound energy has the potential to allow for the pre-natal diagnosis of a whole host of anomalies, **BUT** the case for screening has not in fact been proven."* She called for large multicentre trials to be performed in all types of units, not just the large referral units, so that the reliability of diagnoses could be evaluated. She also made the very valid point that the natural history of many of the minor abnormalities is unknown. The process of further investigations following their discovery can generate a great deal of anxiety.

Maureen Gowland, Consultant Radiologist, Bolton Royal Infimary fears that screening for fetal abnormality by ultrasound scan is in danger of becoming another routine impersonal test and its value needs to be clearly defined. Operators untrained in patient counselling should in her view be discouraged as the anxiety produced by such practice may well outweigh the positive benefits *(Gowland, 1988)*.

This particular screening procedure usually takes place at approximately 20 weeks gestation. However screening programmes vary. Sometimes gestational age is confirmed at 16 weeks when an anomaly scan might be attempted. The fetus is too small at this stage to see all the structures clearly.

Very often ultrasound screening accompanies a maternal serum screening programme when a specimen of maternal serum is taken between 16-20 weeks gestation. These blood tests can be limited to measurement of the alpha-fetoprotein levels alone to assess the woman's risk of having a baby with an open neural tube defect, but may also include measurement of chorionic gonadotrophin and oestrogen levels to assess the risk of a fetus with Down's Syndrome. Just how ultrasound scanning complements this type of screening varies widely. If numbers and economics are not prohibitive, a scan taken prior to commencement of the programme has the advantage that the number of false positive diagnoses are diminished. The size of the fetus in relation to gestational age is ascertained. Multiple pregnancy, signs of uterine bleeding and the presence of fibroids, all of which cause the alpha-fetoprotein levels in the serum to be raised, can be detected or excluded.

In evaluating the results of maternal serum screening for detecting those at risk of carrying a baby with Down's syndrome, Wald *(1992)* reported that the use of ultrasound to confirm or revise gestational age reduces the number of false negative and false positive results, but it is not always possible to scan prior to 16 weeks for this purpose and then offer fetal anomaly screening at 20 weeks.

20 weeks is the optimum time for fetal anomaly screening as the fetus is big enough and developed sufficiently for this to be effective. Selective scanning prior to, or at, 16 weeks for women with uncertain dates is often the programme of choice, followed by the scanning of all women at 20 weeks. This can be achieved perfectly satisfactorily in most units according to Gardosi *(Gardosi, 1993)*.

There are two approaches to a programme of screening for fetal anomalies. 1) Women who are at 'low risk' of having a baby suffering from any chromosomal, genetic or structural abnormality. That is they have no history of having had such a baby themselves, and/or there is no family history of any such problem.

Screening is offered to these women as part of a routine programme, as something that is available to them should they wish to participate. They do not therefore anticipate a problem, although a certain amount of anxiety might be generated because of being offered the test in the first instance. It comes as a great shock should an anomaly be found.

2) The second group comprises the women who are at 'high risk' of having a baby with an abnormality. They have either had a baby with some congenital problem, or have a family history of such a condition. These women seek reassurance from the tests, and seek advice about the correct programme of screening procedures that will suit their particular situation. There is great anxiety during the course of the tests. Finding an abnormality is at least half expected, although it still proves to be a shock. Relief is great if the tests prove to be negative. Within this group are those who have positive results from maternal serum screening.

It is during the second trimester that most women receive a scan. Sonographers are becoming more and more aware of the demands made upon them by performing such detailed examinations of the fetus. Litigation is becoming an increasing threat which is one reason why some sonographers examine the fetus in detail at every scan, regardless of the reason for the investigation. Records of the scan should be made immediately and include all aspects of the examination, plus the signature of the sonographer. It is the records that come under scrutiny in any case that comes before the courts.

The exact nature and details of the 20 week scan for abnormalities will be described in the next chapter.

CHAPTER 8

The Second Trimester Scan – Examination of the Skeleton

The ultrasound examination in the second trimester can form the basis of any further examination that takes place in the pregnancy. It is the ideal time to measure the fetus, confirm or establish gestational age *(Warsof, 1983)*, examine the fetus for anomalies and locate the situation of the placenta in relation to the internal cervical os. The position of a low lying placenta in early pregnancy can change as the pregnancy advances and the lower uterine segment develops.

The examination itself needs to be systematic so that nothing is missed. Most sonographers start with looking at the head and spine. They then proceed to examine the rest of the skeleton, and finally the other systems, namely; cardiac, gastro-intestinal and renal.

The Head and Spine

Having obtained the correct image of the head, the image is frozen and the following dimensions are obtained:-

The bi-parietal diameter (BPD) and the head circumference (HC).

These measurements aid in the confirmation of the gestational age and form a baseline on which future monitoring of growth can be compared.

The anatomy of the head is then examined. The anterior horns of the lateral ventricles can be seen from this image. The distance between the anterior horn of the lateral ventricle and the midline is measured, together with the distance from the midline to the border of the skull. It is expressed in the form of a ratio and is known as the ventricular/hemisphere ratio (V/H ratio). This measurement should be less than 0.5 after 18 weeks gestation, i.e. the distance from the midline to the anterior horn should be less than half the measurement from the midline to the skull border. The position of the posterior horns are measured in the same way. The horns contain the choroid plexus which can be seen clearly from this view.

Cerebrospinal fluid (CSF) is produced by the choroid plexus and circulates through the ventricular system, around the brain and around the spine. Enlargement of the ventricular/hemisphere ratio, means the fetus has hydrocephaly caused by either excess production with slow absorption of the cerebrospinal fluid, or an obstruction in the communicating system.

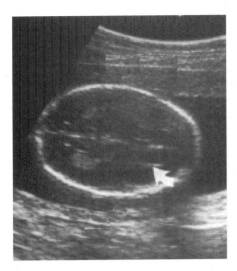

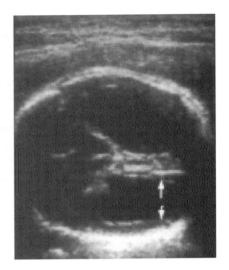

Fig. 8.1 Normal head
arrow indicates ventricular horn

Fig. 8.2 Hydrocephalus - dialated horns
of ventricles indicated by arrows

Interestingly the bi-parietal diameter (BPD) and the head circumference (HC) are not enlarged at this stage in cases of hydrocephaly, although this may develop later in the pregnancy. The brain begins to develop normally but regresses with the accumulation of the fluid as the ventricles enlarge.

Obstructive hydrocephalus is characterised by enlargement of both of the lateral ventricles and the third ventricle, with a normal fourth ventricle. There is in this instance little likelihood of other anomalies. Where the condition is mild with little loss of brain tissue, the insertion of a shunt postnatally is followed by a low mortality rate and intellectual development is good. In severe cases of hydrocephaly associated with destruction of brain tissue, morbidity and mortality rates are high. Isolated hydrocephaly is sometimes sex linked, so the woman might have had a male infant with the condition. In these instances scans should be repeated until 26-28 weeks as the cause, a stenosis of the aqueduct, may present quite late. If the fetus can be identified as a female this is obviously not necessary.

Hydrocephalus is associated with neural tube defects in 60-90% of cases. The enlarged ventricular/hemisphere ratio should therefore alert the sonographer to examine the spine in great detail. In cases of spina-bifida the head is also likely to be 'lemon' shaped.

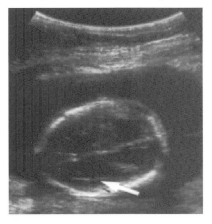

*Fig. 8.3 Lemon-shaped head
arrow indicating dilated ventrical*

Other structures in the head should be examined before looking at the spine. The cavum septum pellucidum, which looks like a little equals sign, is a third of the way along the midline. Its presence excludes holoprosencephaly which is a condition characterised by a single ventricle. The brain has failed to divide into two hemispheres.

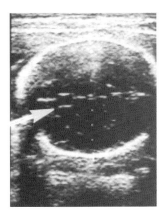
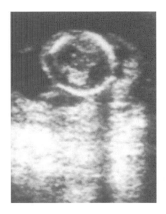

*Fig. 8.4 Normal head
arrow indicates cavum septum
pellucidum*

Fig. 8.5 Holoprosencephaly

Moving the transducer slightly demonstrates the presence of the cerebellum and the midbrain; this too can be measured. A 'banana' shaped cerebellum is another indication of the presence of a neural tube defect. Other causes of an abnormal cerebellum are Dandy Walker Syndrome, a rare condition often associated with other anomalies indicative of Trisomies 18, 21, and 13.

The choroid plexus seen within the ventricular system either side of the midline sometimes contains cysts. The presence of choroid plexus cysts is the source of much controversy. They can be associated with chromosomal abnormalities, in particular trisomy 18, in which case they are usually bilateral and comparatively large. If they are seen on a routine scan they cause a dilemma. Very often, if they are unilateral and small and no other chromosome markers can be identified, a repeat scan after one month will find them reduced in size and eventually they will disappear. One theory is that these are associated with a period of anoxia.

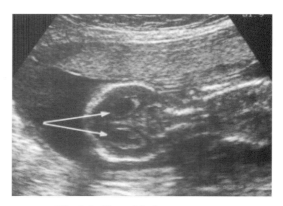

Fig. 8.6 Choroid plexus cysts

A multi-centre study performed in 1993 quotes the risk of a chromosomal abnormality as being 1in 200 following discovery of isolated choroid plexus cysts on routine ultrasound examination in a 'low risk' population. For women over the age of 37years this risk was found to increase to 10% *(Chitty, 1993)*. In the units participating in this study, these findings resulted in a policy of offering karyotyping to all women in whom the cysts had been found on routine ultrasound scan at 18-20 weeks *(Walkinshaw, 1993)*. They were counselled regarding the predicted result. Some feel a more conservative approach is advisable, offering karyotyping only if other anomalies are present at the time of the scan. If the fetus appears in every other aspect to be normal, repeat scanning is offered to monitor the size and hopefully the regression of the cysts *(Twining, 1993)*.

There are other abnomalies of the head that can be diagnosed but they are rare and are probably only seen with any frequency in the large regional centres. Most are referred in the first instance because the sonographer recognises a deviation from the normal, but cannot make a diagnosis.

Microcephaly is not an easy diagnosis to make on ultrasound. It cannot be made on a single examination, but might be suspected if the measurements of the head do not correlate with the other measurements of the fetus. Serial scanning of the head will confirm a slow growth in comparison to the abdominal circumference and the limb lengths. The cause of microcephaly can be difficult to establish; it can be viral, and some cases might be autosomal recessive, but for the majority a cause will never be established.

Neural Tube Defects

The most obvious abnormality which is quite easily diagnosed is absence of the vault of the skull, that is anencephaly. This can be detected from as early as 12-14 weeks gestation. The eyes appear very prominent but the measurements of the head are impossible to obtain due to absence of the vault.

Encephalocele is a defect of the cranial vault in the area of the occiput, although it may be in the frontal, nasal or parietal bones. There is a protusion of the brain through the defect. The sac composed of dura mater and its contents can easily be seen on scan. The fetus is usually microcephalic. It is sometimes associated with polycystic kidneys when it is known as Meckel's sydrome.

Spina bifida

The normal spine appears as two sets of parallel dots which converge to a point at the sacrum where there is a curve upwards in a little flick. The neck end widens at the entrance to the base of the skull. The image obtained should show a skin cover in both the longitudinal and transverse sections.

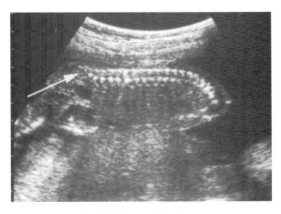

Fig. 8.7 Normal spine
arrow indicates sacral curve

Transversely the ossified bony vertebrae can easily be identified as a ring. Any vertebrae remaining open can be visualised as a V. The most common areas for spina bifida are the cervical area, the lumbar spine or lumbar sacral area. There is splaying of the parallel line at the region of the defect and very often the soft tissue protusion through it,(the sac of the meningocele), can be seen. The maternal serum alpha-fetoprotein level will be high.

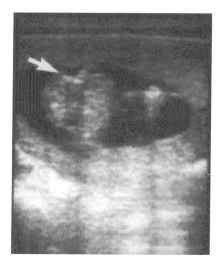 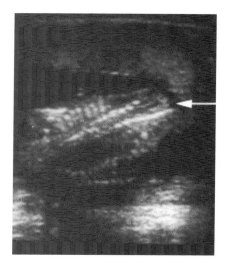

Fig. 8.8 Transverse section of spine arrow indicates neural tube defect

Fig. 8.9 Longitudinal section of spine - arrow indicates splaying of spine at site of defect

Other skeletal abnormalities

Measurement of the femur is a useful parameter in confiming gestational age, together with the bi-parietal diameter (BPD). The measurements obtained should correlate so that the expected date of delivery can be estimated. If there is discrepancy between the femur length and the head measurement, other possibilities should be considered. These include microcephaly, a limb abnormality or a chromosomal abnormality.

All the limbs and also the ribs should then be examined. It is not usual to measure them all unless the woman has a history of some bone defomity, or the femur measurements appear short. Limb deformities fall into the following groups:- absence of part of, or the whole of a limb, absence of a long bone, shortening of the long bones and osteogenesis imperfecta congenita. Extra digits and abnormal positioning of the limbs can also be determined.

A short femur has been associated with Trisomy 21 (Down's Syndrome) *(Lockwood, 1987).*

Marked limb reduction suggests a form of achondroplasia. On examining the chest the ribs may be short, the thorax small and narrow or bell shaped and the abdomen appears large. There are numerous types of this condition, many having a poor prognosis, mainly due to failure of the lungs to develop which is caused by the abnormally narrow chest. When achondroplasia is suspected at the time of the scan the woman should be referred to a centre specialising in this type of condition. It is useful to obtain an accurate family history to assist in the formation of a diagnosis. Some types of achondroplasia are autosomal recessive. Those with achondroplasia which is not complicated by life threatening conditions grow up as dwarfs and are often employed as clowns in the circus. Osteogenesis imperfecta also presents as shortened limbs. In addition the limbs may be deformed due to the presence of fractures.

Absence of a long bone, for example the radius, is often associated with chromosomal abnormalities.

Talipes is detected by examination of the angle of the tibia to the foot. Although it can occur in isolation, it can also be present with other abnormalities and can again be associated with chromosomal abnormalities including Down's syndrome. Rocker bottom feet, extra toes and abnormal positions can also be classed as chromosome markers. Club hands, crossed fingers, extra or absent phalanges are equally suspicious.

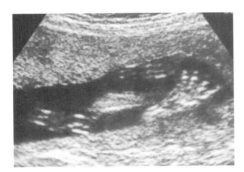 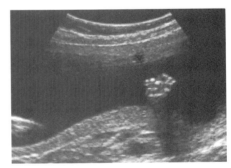

Fig. 8.10 Normal hand   *Fig. 8.11 Abnormal hand – clenched fist and overlapping fingers*

Taken in isolation these minor abnormalities are all probably insignificant, but when seen collectively or associated with other organ defects karyotyping should be considered.

CHAPTER 9

The Second Trimester Scan – Examination of internal organs

After examining the skeleton, the internal structures and the various systems are scanned.

The Abdomen

A cross section of the abdomen is obtained and the abdominal circumference is measured. The section should be almost a perfect circle, where a short section of the umbilical vein can be seen a third of the way across. The fetal stomach is visible to the left and a transverse section of the aorta and the fetal spine opposite to the umbilical vein. This section should be measured to form a baseline for future reference if the growth of the fetus needs to be monitored. It is not a very satisfactory measurement to use when estimating gestational age.

Body Wall Defects

High maternal serum alpha-fetoprotein levels are present in open defects of the fetus. This includes abdominal defects where leakage of body fluids may take place. Ultrasound is very useful, therefore, in making a differential diagnosis in cases of raised maternal serum alpha-fetoprotein. This is very important because unless a cause for the raised maternal serum alpha-fetoprotein is known, counselling of the parents regarding the fetal outcome cannot usefully take place. Whereas a neural tube defect may have a poor prognosis, for some of the other defects causing a raised maternal serum alpha-fetoprotein the prognosis might be entirely different.

Gastroschisis (incidence1:10-15,000) is a condition where the abdominal contents are herniated through a hole in the abdominal wall. They are not enclosed in a sac and the cord is adjacent to the external mass. It is not usually associated with chromosomal defects. Prognosis depends on how much of the abdominal contents are herniated and the size of the hole in the abdominal wall. If it is too small and restricting it can diminish the blood supply to the herniated mass. Prognosis can be good following the appropriate surgery to replace the gut, but feeding problems may continue for some time. If the 'tourniquet' effect of a small hole is severe, gut problems may develop.

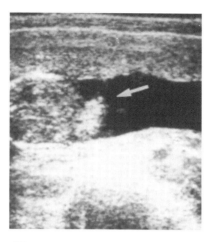

Fig. 9.1 Transverse section of fetal abdomen - herniated loops of bowel indicated by arrow

Exomphalos (incidence 1:5,000) may or may not be associated with raised maternal serum alpha-fetoprotein. In this condition the herniated contents are contained within a membranous sac and the umbilical vessels run through it. It is associated with cardiac defects and chromosomal abnormalities.

Because exomphalos is associated with other perhaps more serious anomalies, it is important that the correct diagnosis is made and that this condition is distinguished from gastroschisis. One of the most important observations is to recognise the presence or absence of a sac around the abdominal contents. Before parents are counselled regarding this condition, karyotyping of the fetus needs to be performed so that the professionals concerned with advising the parents have a more accurate idea of the prognosis . If the condition is isolated the prognosis is usually very good, although it does mean prolonged and repeated surgery for the child

If the bladder has herniated through the abdominal wall, surgery is usually successful, but there can remain kidney and continence problems.

Obstructive Disorders

Other types of anomalies are the obstructive defects, usually associated with polyhydramnios. Just as at delivery copious amounts of liquor alert those present to the possibility of an obstruction in the alimentary system, so its appearance on scan alerts the sonographer in the same way. Absence of the echo free space (see Fig. 9.2) of the stomach together with polyhydramnios should suggest oesophageal atresia. When an associated fistula is present a stomach shadow can be seen, but it is consistently small on repeated scans, so if the polyhydramnios persists the condition should be suspected (incidence 1:5,000).

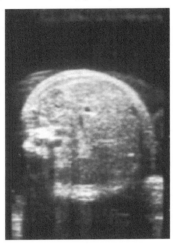

Fig. 9.2 Transverse section of fetal abdomen.

Duodenal atresia presents as a double bubble, that is two stomach shadows, or echo free areas, with the associated polyhydramnios (incidence1:10,000).

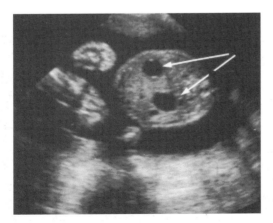

Fig. 9.3 Transverse section of fetal abdomen
illustrating double-bubble

Lower obstructions of the alimentary tract present as an increasing number of echo free areas with varying degrees of polyhydramnios. Associated abnormalities are common, including skeletal and chromosomal conditions. Again, therefore, fetal karyotyping is necessary before a true picture of the fetal condition can be assessed and the parents counselled accordingly.

Chest Abnormalities

Congenital heart disease is quite a common abnormality. Many of the minor defects are not detected until late in life. They are also a marker to other problems, particularly chromosomal defects, the most common being Down's syndrome. The four chambers of the heart should be examined, a cross section of the chest having been obtained. The more serious abnormalities will be detected by obtaining a clear view showing the auricles and the ventricles and the action of the heart valves. It has been suggested that 80% of cardiac abnormalities detected are referred to larger centres because of visualisation of an abnormal four chamber view. According to Lindsey Allan writing in the British Medical Journal in 1986, if all sonographers examined the heart in this way at the routine ultrasound examination, it would result in the detection of over 60% of severe structural abnormalities of the heart which usually present in the first year of life *(Allan, 1986)*. The major blood vessels, in particular the aortic root and the origin of pulmonary artery can be visualised. Women with a history of a congenital heart defect, or who have had a previous baby with such a defect, should be offered a scan at a large referral centre specialising in this type of scanning. The actual diagnosis of this type of defect is not something that can usually be performed by the sonographer in the course of a routine scan. There is a recurrence risk of approximately 3% after the birth of one affected child which rises to 10-15% after the birth of two affected children *(Fowlie, 1991)*.

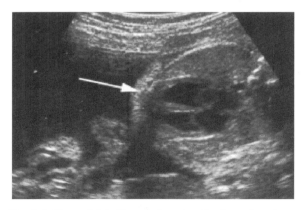

Fig. 9.4 Normal fetal heart showing the four chambers

The lungs can be seen while examining the chest and any cystic spaces identified. Diaphragmatic hernia (incidence1:2,000) is suspected if the echo free area of the stomach is seen adjacent to the heart.

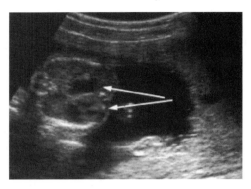

Fig. 9.5 Cross section of the chest - arrows indicate stomach shadow adjacent to the fetal heart

It is sometimes found when the operator is trying to obtain the correct cross section to measure the abdominal circumference. The landmarks are difficult to identify, their position having shifted into the chest area. Sometimes the defect in the diaphragm can be seen. Again this condition can be associated with other abnormalities. If diagnosed ante-natally it improves the prognosis because the place of delivery and the facilities needed to perform immediate surgery on the baby can be arranged. Outcome depends very much on the condition of the lungs; expansion in fetal life may be inhibited because of the limited space in the chest caused by the presence of the abdominal contents resulting in lung hypoplasia. This has led to the development of fetal surgery in utero for this condition in some of the larger centres, having been pioneered in the U.S.A.

Kidney Abnormalities

Oligohydramnios should raise suspicions of kidney anomalies. When it occurs, together with no identifiable bladder, it should immediately alert the sonographer to suspect renal agenesis, polycystic kidneys or kidney aplasia. These women are very difficult to scan because of the oligohydramnios, there being virtually no fluid background to distinguish the image being examined. The textures of the varying tissues merge and the fetus itself is cramped and squashed. These babies very often present as a breech.

Oligohydramnios is also a feature of severe growth retardation of the fetus and differential diagnosis can be very difficult. If there is no evidence of urine production prognosis is poor as many of the associated conditions are incompatible with life.

On finding cysts in the kidney, the sonographer should ascertain whether they are multiple, single, bilateral or unilateral. The kidneys are measured and a differential diagnosis is made. Evidence of urine production by visualisation of a filling and emptying bladder improves any prognosis. In the case of unilateral kidney cysts with good urine production and normal liquor volume, the prognosis is good. All babies who appear to have kidney problems in utero, however minor, need a scan in the post-natal period for a precise diagnosis.

Stricture, or agenesis of the urethra presents as oligohydramnios, but with a greatly distended bladder. The condition of the kidneys should be assessed as back pressure may cause irreparable damage in some instances. In the event of this condition, intrauterine intervention to decompress the renal obstruction has been tried, although this is controversial. Results have proved unsuccessful. Very often these babies have associated chromosomal abnormalities and the outcome is poor *(Gibbon and Hayward, 1991)*.

Routine ultrasound scanning often reveals anomalies of the kidney, for example renal cysts, or hydronephrosis of one or both kidneys. Mild dilatation of the renal pelves may be associated with chromosomal disorders. The actual diagnosis is not easy unless a definite cause for these anomalies can also be seen. It is therefore left until the baby is born when a further scan and examination of the urine and urinary output enables a diagnosis to be made.

Sometimes nothing abnormal is detected despite the antenatal picture. In these instances the infant is rescanned after a period of six weeks. It has been suggested that a further scan after a similar period is advisable. Providing these results are normal, the parents can be reassured. It does mean, of course, that this scenario generates a great deal of unnecessary anxiety for the family. Just occasionally, however, serious kidney disease is averted because the paediatrician has been alerted about a potential problem due to the prenatal screening by ultrasound scan. An example of this is when mild dilatation of the kidney pelvis has been identified. Occasionally this leads to severe kidney damage if left undetected and the cause is not investigated.

The Umbilical Cord

It is possible to count the vessels in the cord by obtaining a cross section. There should be two arteries and one vein. If only one artery is visualised, abnormalities of the renal tract should be suspected.

Fetal Hydrops or Hydrops Fetalis

Fetal hydrops is associated with rhesus isoimmunisation, but this condition is now comparatively rare. It is more commonly associated with non-immune hydrops. Fetal hydrops is easily recognised by the presence of ascites and/or pleural effusions, together with skin oedema. There are a variety of causes, including cardiovascular chromosomal conditions. It may be the result of infection, for example, cytomegalovirus. The prognosis is usually poor, but the condition has been known to resolve spontaneously.

Sexing the Fetus

The fetal genitals should be examined. Some sonographers reveal the sex to the parents, if the parents do not see for themselves. Units may have a policy of not divulging the sex to the family. It has been reported that abortion has been sought by some parents if the fetus is not the sex of their choice. Hydroceles can be diagnosed. They can be associated with more serious anomalies, but this is unusual.

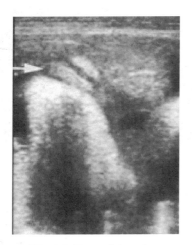

Fig. 9.6 Normal female -
arrow indicates labia majora

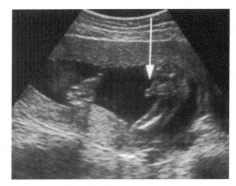

Fig. 9.7 Normal male -
arrow indicates male genitalia

Locating the Placenta

The position of the placenta with particular reference to its relationship to the lower segment and the internal cervical os is noted. Again this is useful as a screening procedure. A seemingly low lying placenta at this stage does not mean that it will remain so. Placental examination and position will be discussed in a later chapter.

Fetal Attitude and Behaviour

While such a detailed scan is taking place it is quite easy to observe fetal movement and fetal behaviour. Thumb sucking, eye rolling, as well as limb and body movements are a normal occurrence so, as well as assuring the sonographer that the fetus is behaving normally, the woman and her partner are able to see their baby moving about on the screen. This is tremendously reassuring and a source of great joy to all concerned. If abnormalities are found the woman and her partner become very aware that something is wrong even if nothing is said by the sonographer. Body language, concern, shock and the increased concentration of the operator convey this to the woman very quickly. It is essential, therefore, that before embarking on such an examination as this, a fool proof back up system with obstetricians and possibly paediatricians is available. In this way, expert advice and support can be given immediately and an accurate prognosis of the condition can be given to the prospective parents as soon as possible after a diagnosis has been made.

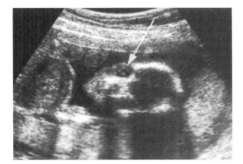

Fig. 9.8 Fetal eye

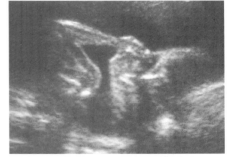

Fig. 9.9 Thumb-sucking

Termination of the pregnancy should not be seen as the only option for any abnormality. As well as discussion with paediatricians with regard to potential problems that may be encountered, information regarding the support services available for any particular condition should also be to hand, should the prospective parents decide to bring up what may be a handicapped child.

CHAPTER 10

Ultrasound Markers of Anomalies

In the previous two chapters a detailed account of the second trimester scan has been described, with particular reference to any anomalies, as this is the usual format for a scan performed at this time. As has already been argued, it is difficult to perform a scan without seeing obvious abnormalities, so the sonographer really cannot scan a woman just to confirm or establish gestational age of the fetus without there being the possibility that an abnormality might be discovered.

It has also been suggested that there are various markers, or signs that might be observed while performing this scan, that might be indicative of serious anomalies. On the other hand these markers might be of little significance.

It is useful, however, when one or two of these markers have been observed, to have some knowledge as to what the potential problems might be. Taken in isolation, some of the minor abnormalities can cause parents a great deal of anxiety unnecessarily. One such example might be talipes, or perhaps an extra digit. A fetal karyotype is essential to confirm suspicions of a chromosomal disorder, but this is usually only performed when more than one marker has been identified and there are strong suspicions of more serious problems. Sometimes the defect is a major problem in itself. An example of this might be exomphalus.

The most expedient way of performing a fetal karyotype is by taking a specimen of cord blood which can be obtained by cordocentesis. A specimen of fetal blood is withdrawn from the cord, under direct ultrasound surveillance. The result is usually available within a day or two. This service is not always available at the smaller district maternity units because of the lack of expertise in performing the technique.

After amniocentesis fetal cells in the amniotic fluid are examined for karyotyping. It takes three or four weeks to obtain a result. Because the results take this long, amniocentesis at this stage of the pregnancy ie. 18-20 weeks gestation is not ideal. If an abnormality is confirmed, the parents could be contemplating termination of the pregnancy at 23-24 weeks gestation.

Ideally, observation of markers of chromosome abnormality at the 20 weeks scan should be followed up at a large referral centre where a second opinion can be obtained and immediate cordocentesis carried out, if deemed to be necessary.

To some parents further investigations plus the possibility of terminating a pregnancy is unacceptable, particularly if the markers are very minor and may be of no clinical significance. They therefore choose to continue the pregnancy regardless of the outcome. What should be a joyous time looking forward to the birth of their baby becomes a very anxious wait. Others are prepared to go ahead with further investigations, wishing to know of any problems they might have to face, but are unwilling to contemplate termination of the pregnancy. They must have this option.

The following observations are signs, or markers of more serious disease that might be seen while performing a routine scan. Indication is given about their significance.

Polyhydramnios
This is present in a number of abnormalities, but most particularly in neural tube defects and obstructive disorders of the alimentary tract.

It can also be present in the pregnancy of the diabetic woman and in multiple pregnancies.

Oligohydramnios
This is a present in the following conditions
 1) the kidneys of the fetus are not producing urine, or the fetal kidneys are absent. It is therefore a significant feature of abnormalities of the renal tract, particularly multicystic disease of the kidney and renal agenesis or dysplasia.

2) severe growth retardation of the fetus causes less urine to be produced, so although oligohydramnios may be present, differential diagnosis is important.

CHROMOSOMAL ABNORMALITIES

Features of trisomy 13

This condition was described by Patau in 1960. The incidence is quoted as being 1:5000 *(Twining, 1991)*. The prognosis is poor. Most of the typical features are seen in the head and neck and include:-

Holoprosencephaly, agenesis of the corpus callosum and sometimes hydrocephalus.
Clefts of the lip and palate are sometimes present, as are low set ears.
Other rarer abnormalities that can be a feature include renal tract anomalies, heart defects and rockerbottom feet.
Severe growth retardation might be the first indication of a problem.

Features of trisomy 18 (Edward's Syndrome)

The incidence of this condition is said to be 1:3000 The prognosis is poor.
Abnormalities include:-
Rocker-bottom feet and flexion of the fingers with overlapping. This is associated with radial aplasia and club hands.

When examining the head the sonographer might find evidence of micrognathia, clefts of the lip and palate, choroid plexus cysts and occasionally hydrocephaly.

Diaphragmatic hernia, heart defects and abdominal defects are sometimes present.

Again growth retardation is the feature that might draw the sonographer's attention to further problems..

Trisomy 21 Down's Syndrome

The overall incidence is said to be 1-3: 3000 It is age related, the incidence being greater with increasing maternal age. *(Twining, 1991)*

Markers for this syndrome can be any one or a combination of the following:-

A short femur length for the gestational age, in comparison to measurements of the head.

A thick nuchal fold. This is the pad of fat at the back of the neck. It is measured at the same time as the other measurements of the head, and is taken from the skin surface to the outer edge of the occipital bone. If it measures more than 6mm it is abnormal.

There is hypoplasia of the middle phalynx of the 5th finger. Dilatation of the renal pelves, duodenal atresia and cardiac defects are common.

Splaying of the toes may be observed.

Features of Turner's Syndrome, XO or absence of one of the X chromosomes

The incidence is said to be 1:5000.

The characteristic marker for this syndrome is cystic hygroma at the back of the neck, often accompanied by hydrops. If other abnormalities are present prognosis is poor, but the outlook is good if the fetus survives until term. These children are infertile.

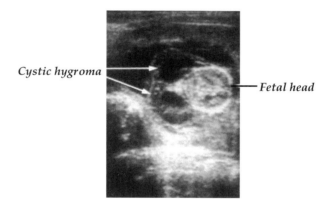

Cystic hygroma — Fetal head

Fig. 10.1 Cystic hygroma associated with Turner's Syndrome

Diagnosis of an abnormality is a disastrous experience for the parents. They will need alot of support in coming to a decision about whether or not to have their pregnancy terminated, if this is an option open to them. Termination is usually offered in cases of chromosomal abnormality and many of the structural defects.

As soon as an abnormality is suspected the parents should be informed. The tension created by the sonographer as he/she concentrates on coming to a diagnosis, once an abnormality is suspected, is soon felt by the woman and her partner. If at all possible they should be given time to come to terms with the diagnosis before they have to make decisions about future action.

In discussing the counselling necessary when informing parents about the diagnosis, Anthony (1984) states *"the disagreeable meaning of this highly personal information affects the processing of the information by the counsellees so that either they distort its meaning or are highly selective in their attention————Therefore it is important to determine whether information is being remembered and integrated for decision making"*

The big problem at this stage of the pregnancy is the time factor. Even so parents should not be rushed into making decisions. Parents deciding to have their pregnancy terminated should be put in touch with the organisation called Support Around Termination for Fetal Abnormality (S.A.T.F.A.). Sara Kenyon identified the need to follow up these women because of their special problems and the guilt feelings associated with the fact that they have not lost their baby spontaneously, but have actively taken a decision which has been responsible for the baby's death *(Kenyon, 1988)*. S.A.T.F.A. branches have been started throughout the country and these families can seek support and advice from mothers who have gone through a similar experience.

Parents deciding to go ahead with the pregnancy and give birth to a handicapped child need the special support necessary to come to terms with that fact. They can also be put in touch with appropriate support groups. It is the job of the health care professionals to help and support them in whatever decision they make.

CHAPTER 11

Ultrasound Scanning in the Third Trimester of Pregnancy

Up until the early 1980s it was the usual practice to scan women in the third trimester of pregnancy as a screening procedure to check for abnormal fetal growth.

Growth retardation of the fetus is the most common congenital abnormality seen in the neonate. The growth retarded fetus is more likely to be stillborn *(Usher and Mclean, 1974)*, to suffer from fetal distress in labour *(Lin, 1980)*, and to be at risk of neonatal problems, including developmental disorders *(Fitzhardinge and Steven, 1972)* which may subsequently lead to low intelligence quotient or even mental handicap.

Recent research has indicated that there is a definite link between the growth retarded fetus and diseases in adult life, in particular cardiovascular diseases and diabetes mellitus *(Barker, 1993)*.

However, not all small babies are growth retarded. Some are small because they are genetically determined to be small. They represent the lower end of the normal range, are perfectly proportioned and do not experience the problems associated with growth retardation.

Symmetrical growth retardation

Other small babies, again correctly proportioned, are termed symmetrically growth retarded (see chapter 5). Babies in this group have usually been subjected to some environmental factor that has caused problems of growth. Causes include babies suffering from chromosomal abnormalities, or intra-uterine infections such as toxoplasmosis and cytomegalovirus. Babies of mothers who are substance abusers, smoke, or have been exposed to ionising radiation also come into this group. Fetal alcohol syndrome is also a cause of a small fetus.

For fetuses suffering from symmetrical growth retardation, a karyotype should be considered, or a scan to look specifically for markers of chromosome abnormalities.

Advice can be given to women with a fetus suffering from symmetrical growth retardation on the environmental factors that might be affecting the fetus, for example smoking and drinking habits. Measurement of the blood flow in maternal and/or fetal vessels should be considered.

Assymetrical growth retardation

Babies with asymmetrical growth retardation have a head size equivalent to their age but they appear thin and look as if they have been starved, which of course they have, as this type of growth deficiency is associated with placental insufficiency. As well as being starved of nutrition they are also starved of oxygen and may well suffer from irreparable brain damage. In some instances, if the condition is unnoticed, it can cause perinatal death.

Asymmetrical growth retarded fetuses might benefit from a biophysical profile, including liquor volume measurements and measurement of the blood flow in maternal and/or fetal vessels.

When born these babies often suffer from hypoglycaemia, hypothermia and hypocalcaemia which can again have long lasting effects on the development of the child.

Small for gestational age infants have birth weights under the 10th. centile for their gestational age. Decisions as to whether they fall into this category should only be made after considering their ethnic origin and the existent population from which they derive. Birthweight standards vary according to these factors *(Wilcox, 1993)*.

Babies suffering from intra-uterine growth retardation need not be small for gestational age. In order to monitor fetal growth it is important to scan before 24weeks gestation so that a base line can be established. A fetus scanned in the second trimester with measurements at the upper end of the range, born with measurements at the lower end, would seemingly have suffered some form of growth retardation, while remaining within normal parameters for that gestational age.

The Macrosomic Fetus

The macrosomic fetus also causes problems, particularly at birth. Cephalo-pelvic disproportion can occur, as can shoulder dystocia. Both may result in perinatal death. Damage to the brachial plexus, resulting in paralysis of the face and arms, can also be the result of severe shoulder dystocia.

Lower segment caesarean section may be necessary if the fetus is too large to pass through the female pelvis, with the associated risks of anaesthesia. Many such babies are born to mothers with diabetes mellitus, thus this condition should be assessed and any polyhydramnios identified. In measuring the growth, these fetuses will have a growth pattern above the 90th centile.

As in the small fetus, it is essential when observing all growth patterns that the initial measurements that form the baseline are obtained before 24 weeks gestation.

Measurement of Fetal Growth

Measurements used to plot the growth of the fetus have already been described, but those most commonly used are the head circumference and the abdominal circumference most commonly expressed in a ratio, HC/AC.

Routine screening by ultrasound to observe fetal growth patterns is not usually performed these days. Research performed at King's College Hospital compared measuring the symphysis fundal height (SFH) by tape-measure with measuring the abdominal circumference by ultrasound revealed that the much simpler method of measuring the symphysis fundal height by tape measure was equally sensitive in predicting the small fetus *(Pearce & Campbell, 1983)*.

For this reason ultrasound examination to monitor fetal growth is usually restricted to those groups of women who fall into the 'high risk' category. These should include women with a poor obstetric history, for example stillbirth or previous babies suffering from intra-uterine growth retardation. Women suffering from pregnancy-induced hypertension, diabetes mellitus, sickle cell disease, essential hypertension or cardiac disease. Women who are heavy smokers, alcoholics or drug abusers might also benefit from a scan to monitor fetal growth. Multiple pregnancy is also included in the high risk category. A single scan in the third trimester for women in these groups will not necessarily detect abnormal patterns of growth. Serial scanning at four weekly intervals is usually performed, in some instances every two weeks. In this way fetal growth can be charted in graph form and is easily monitored.

The rest of the pregnant population are usually scanned on request should the symphysis fundal height appear abnormal. These women, having been told that there is a suspicion of a growth problem, should not be left to await results of their scan until the next clinic visit because of the anxiety that this causes. They should be told the results during the scan or immediately afterwards.

Sometimes obstetricians who are anxious about the growth of the fetus request frequent ultrasound examinations at less than two weekly intervals. Such frequent ultrasound examinations are not reliable and are likely to give a false picture of the state of the fetus. The known risk of human error in measurement is greater than a normal weekly growth increment. Therefore weekly scans can indicate a normal growth pattern when there is no growth or they can indicate reduced growth when in fact it is normal. It is not safe practice to perform, or request, scans on women at such frequent intervals. Sonographers should be able to question this practice. There are other clinical parameters that can be examined.

The biophysical profile of the fetus

This is an observational study of the fetal behaviour over a period of 30 minutes, as described by Manning in 1981. Several parameters are used to produce a score which is said to indicate the state of fetal well-being. The parameters used can be modified from those that Manning originally used, but are based on the following:-

Heart rate and its variability; fetal movement, including gross body movement as well as limb and facial movements; fetal breathing movements; fetal tone as demonstrated by clenching fists and extending the fingers or toes; tongue movement and eye rolling. The liquor volume is usually assessed, the presence of more than one pocket of over 1cm in depth is requisite.

Since the study by Proud and Grant in 1987, the texture of the placenta can also be used as an indication of the state of the fetus in conjunction with the above. Early maturation of the placenta is a possible indication of fetal compromise.

Fetal Weight Estimation

Fetal weight estimation is not a parameter used in screening for growth abnormalities, but it can be useful in certain instances including the following:-

a) Breech presentation, when the method of delivery is under consideration.

b) Maternal diabetes, if poorly controlled and macrosomia of the fetus is suspected. Vaginal delivery may be difficult if the fetus is very large.

c) When intra-uterine growth retardation is thought to be severely compromising the fetus.

d) In instances of multiple pregnancy, again to decide upon the management of the delivery.

e) Pre-term labour, to make a decision about whether to suppress the labour or let it continue. It is usual to let labour continue if the fetus weighs more than 2.5kg. Babies weighing 2.5kg or more can be quite safely managed on the special care baby unit. Smaller babies are best managed in an intensive care unit. If such facilities are not available locally the best course of action is to transfer the mother before delivery to a hospital with a neonatal intensive care unit. The risks associated with the transfer of a sick baby at birth are then avoided.

Location of Placental Site

A frequent request for a scan in the third trimester is to establish the cause of vaginal bleeding. The placental site is usually established at the second trimester scan. Placentae thus demonstrated to be encroaching on the lower segment are rescanned in the third trimester to see if they have 'moved'. This so called movement of the placenta occurs due to the growth of the uterus and the development of the lower segment. The relationship between the lower edge of the placenta to the internal cervical os therefore alters. It is also important to establish whether, if the position of the placenta is considered to be borderline, it is situated on the anterior or posterior wall of the uterus. Whereas an anterior placenta which slightly encroaches into the lower segment may not impede vaginal delivery, a posterior placenta sometimes obstructs the descent of the presenting part. A placenta positioned adjacent to, or across the internal os necessitates delivery by caesarean section. In all cases of placenta praevia there is a risk of placental separation and bleeding.

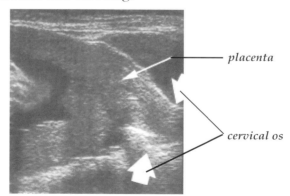

placenta

cervical os

Fig. 11.1 Placenta situated over cervical os

When the placental site is known requests for repeated scanning to locate the site every time the woman bleeds should be discouraged. The only indication for repeated scanning in cases of placenta praevia is to assess fetal growth, because persistent disturbance of the placental site might compromise the fetus. If the woman remains undelivered by 36 weeks gestation, a repeat scan should be performed then *(Chudleigh, 1983)*. If it remains a grade 2, 3 or 4 placenta praevia, elective lower segment caesarean section should be planned.

Placental abruption is suspected when a woman presents with continuous abdominal pain, sometimes accompanied by vaginal bleeding. It is not an easy diagnosis to make but very often ultrasound is requested to ascertain the presence of a retroplacental clot. Small clots cannot be seen and large areas of retroplacental bleeding cause fetal death, so the only place for ultrasound under these circumstances is to assess the condition of the fetus and perhaps, sadly, confirm absence of a fetal heart beat.

CHAPTER 12

Doppler Ultrasound

It is interesting to delve into the history of how the mysteries of fetal circulation came to be understood. As early as 1774 it was hypothesised that oxygenated blood was transported from the placenta to the left side of the heart. In the 1930s the circulatory system was examined in animals but it was not until the 1950s that the route of arterial and venous blood in the fetus was established. Work done in 1959 by Satomura, who investigated the blood flow velocities of the fetus by the Doppler principal, has made it possible to study fetal blood flow.

The Principles of Doppler Ultrasound

A vibrating crystal transmits a beam of ultrasound into the body. Wherever a structure is encountered (or boundary) some of this electrical energy is transferred back. This energy, when received from a boundary that is still, remains at the same frequency, but when it encounters a moving boundary it undergoes a frequency change. This is known as the Doppler shift. The frequency increases or decreases according to whether the movement is towards or away from the source of energy.

In continuous wave Doppler there are two crystals, one emitting the energy and the other receiving it back. The frequencies between the two are compared. An example of a continuous wave Doppler machine is the fetal heart detector. In this machine the movement of the fetal heart is produced as sound which is amplified so that it can easily be heard.

Pulsed wave Doppler involves just one crystal which both emits the energy and receives the echo in short pulses.

The blood flow can therefore be measured through a vessel by this method, provided the diameter of the vessel is known at the site where the flow is measured. Using the Doppler shift principle blood flow velocities can be measured over a stated period of time. Some of the energy outputs on pulsed wave systems use very high levels and, because some of the measurements, particularly of small fetal vessels, are difficult to obtain this method is infrequently used.

Continuous wave Doppler is the method most commonly used. It compares the velocity of the blood during systole to that at the end of diastole. End diastolic flow is generally accepted to be an indication of peripheral resistance. The area of particular interest as far as this is concerned in monitoring fetal well being is the assessment of resistance to blood flow in the placental villus vascular bed.

Vessels on both sides of the placenta can be studied, for example, the umbilical artery or vein, or even the fetal aorta or carotid arteries. The maternal vessels usually examined are the uterine arteries or one of its branches. Nicolaides demonstrated that absence of end diastolic frequencies in the umbilical artery of the fetus was a sign of fetal hypoxia (Nicolaides, 1988). He suggested, therefore, that measurement of the blood flow in the fetal umbilical artery was a more efficient way of diagnosing the fetus who is becoming hypoxic, rather than relying on measurement of growth. The compromised fetus that does not show signs of growth retardation will not then be missed.

Prior to this Trudinger (1985) studied the use of continuous wave Doppler ultrasound on the maternal vessels and the fetal umbilical artery in mothers with severe hypertension. He demonstrated the association between an abnormal uterine artery waveform and abnormal umbilical artery waveforms. Both were associated with obliteration of the small arteries and arterioles in the tertiary villi of the placenta. He also suggested that these findings greatly improve the management of the high risk fetus because detection of fetal compromise would happen earlier than relying on measurement of fetal growth.

Two conditions are of particular interest:-

1) the failure of the cytotrophoblast to invade the spiral arteries of the myometrium which occurs at approximately 16-20 weeks gestation and

2) the development of acute atherosis in the maternal vessels.

Both these conditions are associated with increased vascular resistance which are significant features of intra-uterine growth retardation and pre-eclampsia.

These conditions can be identified by measurement of the diastolic blood flow velocities in the uterine arterial system. Problems may be identified before they produce clinical symptoms. It might therefore be able to predict the fetus that is at risk of compromise.

It could be considered good practice to use Doppler ultrasound as a routine procedure to monitor fetal well being, so that intervention at a suitable moment could possibly prevent death of the hypoxic fetus, or at least prevent some cases of handicap following fetal hypoxia.

Tyrell et al, *(1990)* compared routine selective use of Doppler ultrasound and biophysical profiling in high risk pregnancies. The study was carried out on fetuses already identified as at risk of growth retardation or death. A normal Doppler waveform was associated with a normal neonatal outcome. A persistent abnormal scoring in the biophysical profile was always associated with absence of end diastolic flow. Measurement of blood flow proved to be a more efficient method of monitoring the at risk fetus, outcome being improved when this method was used.

A subsequent study performed in 1993 investigating the possible use of routine Doppler ultrasound in a low risk population came to the conclusion that the benefits to this group were negligible *(Tyrell, 1993)*.

It is not usual practice in most maternity units to offer routine Doppler ultrasound to every pregnant woman,- indeed not all units have the facilities. It is a useful facility to have in the larger centres however, where a high proportion of women are referred because they are considered to be at 'high risk'. Measurement of blood flow in the maternal vessels at the 20 week scan, although recommended at one stage following the study by Nicolaides, is therefore not the normal procedure in most instances.

CHAPTER 13

Invasive Procedures under Ultrasound Guidance

Until the technology of ultrasound came to be used in obstetrics in the 1970s, the only invasive procedure that was performed with any frequency was amniocentesis which was performed 'blind'.

The use of ultrasound has made such procedures much safer because the area where the needle or cannulae should be directed can actually be pin-pointed. It has also enabled information about the state of the fetus to become more available. In all probability the use of invasive procedures has increased, because of the advent of ultrasound. Ultrasound, together with the other biochemical screening tests on the maternal serum, can identify the possibility of abnormalities of the fetus which can lead to the need for further investigation. Further investigation often necessitates the use of invasive procedures.

Amniocentesis

This is the most common invasive procedure of the fetal environment. Fetal epithelial cells removed from the amniotic fluid are cultured and karyotyped. It is also a procedure used in the management of rhesus iso-immunisation of the fetus and in assessing the lecithin sphingomyelin ratio in the fetal lungs, when early induction or delivery is anticipated. Ultrasound scan determines the placental site so that it can be avoided if possible. Confirmation of gestational age of the fetus together with its viability is checked.

Before amniocentesis is started, some clinicians administer a small amount of local anaesthetic to the skin, before introducing the spinal needle, but others consider this 'just another prick' and feel it to be unnecessary. A suitable pool of liquor is identified and a 20-22g spinal needle is guided along the line of the transducer into it. Approximately 20 ml. of liquor is removed. Following the procedure the fetal heart is checked and the woman shown her moving fetus on the screen. Rhesus negative women are given 250iu of anti D serum intramuscularly.

First trimester amniocentesis can now be performed using the same method because a new technique of filtration has been developed. Smaller amounts of liquor are obtained and then filtered to remove the fetal cells. A small study has been performed in Northern Ireland to see if removing a significant amount of fluid as early as 10-13 weeks gestation causes any orthopaedic or respiratory problems in the neonate. The results were compared with a group having had amniocentesis at the more usual gestational age of 16 weeks. There was no significant difference between the two groups *(Dornan, 1993)*. Early amniocentesis is gaining in favour over chorionic villus sampling which is the other test sometimes performed in the first trimester for fetal karyotype. One advantage of early amniocentesis is that a sample of the fluid can also be tested for alpha-fetoprotein. This negates the need for maternal serum screening at a later date with the possibility of facing a late termination of the pregnancy for neural tube defect.

Risks of amniocentesis

These include spontaneous abortion, premature rupture of membranes and intrauterine infection. The risk factor of abortion is said to be 0.5%-1% *(Tabor 1986)*.

Chorionic Villus Sampling (CVS)

This is the technique of removing a small sample of the chorionic villi that surround the gestational sac until approximately 12-14 weeks of the pregnancy. Samples of placental tissue can, in theory, be taken at any stage of the pregnancy, but chorionic villus sampling is usually considered to be a technique performed in the first trimester when a karyotype of the fetus is required.

The villi can be obtained from either the abdominal route, when the technique is the same as that of amniocentesis, or from the vaginal route, having placed the woman in the lithotomy position. A small amount of tissue is aspirated and examined to make sure villi are present.

Because of the nature of the tissue examined, results are available much sooner, in days rather than weeks. Occasionally the results can pose problems, for example in the presence of mosaicism, necessitating a repeat procedure, although as cytogenetic techniques have improved, this has become rare.

Risks of chorionic villus s ampling

In 1991 a European randomised trial reported a significantly higher risk of spontaneous abortion than that following amniocentesis. If performed by experienced hands this risk is much reduced. Figures quoted range from 2%-5%.

An increased incidence of limb and facial abnormalities in babies has been reported. For these reasons its popularity has declined and it should only be used for women at a risk exceeding 1:4 of having a child with a chromosomal defect. The number of women subjecting themselves to chorionic villus sampling or first trimester amniocentesis is likely to rise in view of the increase in the number of the genetic bases of inherited diseases that are becoming known. Women having had chorionic villus sampling also need to be offered maternal serum screening for alpha-fetoprotein levels at 16 weeks gestation. Chorionic villus sampling cannot predict a risk factor for neural tube defects.

The great advantage of chorionic villus sampling is, of course, that it is performed in the first trimester and the results become known with little delay. For women at high risk of having a baby with a chromosomal or genetic defect it is to be preferred to mid trimester amniocentesis even though the risks of abortion are greater, because the wait until 16weeks itself can be very stressful. There is added stress if the woman is able to feel fetal movement before the results of any screening test are known.

Fetal blood sampling

A sample of fetal blood can be obtained from 16 weeks gestation. The site chosen is usually the placental end of the cord, and the technique is the same as that for amniocentesis, except that the needle used is heparinised. 2ml of fetal blood are withdrawn. Karyotyping takes two to three days. It is the test of choice after 20 weeks gestation because the results are available within a few days and thus terminations of pregnancy, if required, can be carried out earlier than if the mother had an amniocentesis. If there is some fetal anomaly the fetus is very often sick by the latter part of the second or the third trimester *(Maxwell, 1991)*. Reasons for fetal blood sampling include the following:-

The observation of chromosome markers on ultrasound scan.
Failed amniocentesis or inconclusive results.
Management of non-immune hydrops.
Investigation and management of Rhesus iso-immunisation.
Prenatal diagnosis of haemoglobinopathies.
Investigations and management of intra-uterine growth retardation.

Fetoscopy

This is not often performed as the techniques described above have improved the diagnosis of a great many of the genetic diseases. It is not usually necessary to directly visualise the fetus or obtain a muscle and/or skin biopsy because this test has been superseded by karyotyping of fetal cells from placental tissue or fetal blood. Many of the conditions can now be diagnosed by fetal blood sampling, or alternatively, visualisation is now often possible by ultrasound as the resolution of the machinery has greatly improved in recent years. The risk to the fetus of introducing an endoscope into the uterus is recorded as being 5%. Introduction of an endoscope through the cervix to examine the developing embryo has also largely been superseded by the advent of the ultrasound vaginal probe.

Fetal Therapy

Fetal surgery is still in the experimental stage, although in the United States of America the results of such procedures are improving. The conditions which produce the best results are those that would probably have the worst prognosis if nothing was attempted. One such condition is diaphragmatic hernia which, if left until term, would render the fetal lungs hypoplastic. The prognosis is therefore poor. Repair of this condition during fetal life has had limited success in the U.S.A. Other conditions for which fetal surgery is sometimes performed are hydrocephalus and renal tract obstruction. Both have had limited success, probably due to the fact that these babies usually have other underlying problems, or the damage already caused by the condition is irreparable.

The number and the extent of invasive procedures is constantly changing as advances in genetics and other diagnostic procedures are developing.

Conclusion

The use of technology in obstetrics has completely revolutionised care in the last decade and ultrasound is responsible for some of the major changes. Like most technology used in this field it has been abused. It seems that many clinicians regard ultrasound as the tool able to provide an answer to every problem. Ultrasound is often the first line of investigation when diagnoses of obstetric problems are made. In some instances women can find themselves being scanned at frequent intervals for a variety of reasons, for example to monitor growth of the fetus, to localise a placenta, or to establish the presenting part, each bearing no relation to the other, and none yielding a significant answer to her problems.

Because of this sonographers should, when scanning pregnant women, examine every feature of the fetus and its environment in the shortest possible time, so that frequent scans for a variety of reasons are not necessary.

Sonographers should also learn to say no if the request seems inappropriate or the request has already been answered on a previous occasion.

Ultrasound scanning cannot give the answer to all problems. It is not the crystal ball that some clinicians like to think it is. It is up to all obstetricians, general practitioners and midwives to familiarise themselves with the technology so that its value can be fully utilised, but it should not be over used or abused.

This book is not meant to be used for those wishing to use the technology. Techniques of using ultrasound have not been described. It is not a text book for sonographers, but a guide to those practitioners wishing to understand its use in obstetrics so that it can be used when appropriate to its full advantage. Practitioners wishing to become ultrasonographers require specialised training, and need to refer to text books describing the physics and use thereof in much greater detail. There is no place for the casual scanner and scanning without training in the technique is unsafe.

I make no apology for quoting Jennett(1984) once again when he said *"High technology medicine is inappropriately deployed if it is unnecessary, (because the desired objective can be achieved by simpler means) unsuccessful, (because the patient has a condition too advanced to respond to treatment) unsafe, (because the possible complications outweigh the possible benefits) unkind, (because the quality of life after rescue is not good enough, or long enough to justify the intervention) or unwise (because it diverts resources from activities that would yield greater benefits).*

References

Chapter 1

Hall, M.H. (1991). "Health of pregnant women". *British Medical Journal*,Vol. 303, pp. 460-2.

United Kingdom Central Council for Nursing, Midwifery and Health Visiting (1993). Midwives Rules, London. p. 21.

Chapter 2

Andrews, M., Webster, M., Fleming, J. and McNay, M. (1987). "Ultrasound exposure time in routine obstetric scanning". *British Journal of Obstetrics and Gynaecology*, Vol. 94, pp. 843-46.

Bakketag, L., Eik-Nes, S.H., Jacobsen, G., Ulsten, M.K., Brodtkorb, C.J., Balstad, P., Eriksen, B.C. and Jorgensen, N.P. (1984). Randomised controlled trial of ultrasonographic screening in pregnancy. *Lancet*, ii, pp. 207-11.

British Medical Ultrasound Society (B.M.U.S) (1993). Secretary's Report,CASE. *B.M.U.S. Bulletin,* May.

Cartwright, R.A., McKinney, P.A., Birch, J.M., Hartley, A.L. *et al.* (1984). "Ultrasound examinations in pregnancy and childhood cancer". *Lancet*, 11, pp. 999-1000.

Duck, F.A., Starritt, H.C., Haar ter, G.R., Lunt, M.J. (1990). "Surface heating of diagnostic ultrasound transducers". *British Journal of Radiology*, Vol. 62, No. 743, pp.1005-13.

Evans, T. (1992). "Safety Issues". *British Medical Ultrasound Society. Bulletin*, August, No. 66, p. 4.

Haar ter, G.R. and Daniels, S. (1981). "Evidence for ultrasonically induced cavitation in vivo". *Physics in Medicine and Biology*, Vol. 26, pp. 1145-49.

Haar ter, G.R., Daniels, S., Eastaugh, K.C. and Hill, C.R. (1982). "Ultrasonically induced cavitation in vivo". *British Journal of Cancer,* Vol. 45, Supplement *v,* pp. 151-55.

Jennett, B. (1984). "High technology medicine". Nuffield Provincial Hospitals Trust, London, pp. 133-34.

Kinnear Wilson, L.M. and Waterhouse, J.A.H. (1984). "Obstetric ultrasound and childhood malignancy". *Lancet* 2, pp. 997-99.

Kremkau, F.W. (1983). "Biological effects and possible hazards". *Clinical Obstetrics and Gynaecology*, Vol.10, pp.395-405.

Liebeskind, D., Bases, R., Mendez, F., Elequin, F. and Koenigsberg, M. (1979). "Sister chromatid exchanges in human lymphocytes after exposure to diagnostic ultrasound". *Science*, Vol. 205, pp. 1273-75.

MacIntosh, I.J.C. and Davey, D.A. (1970). "Chromosome abnormalities induced by an ultrasonic fetal pulse detector". *British Medical Journal*, Supplement iv, pp. 92-93.

MacIntosh, I.J.C. and Davey, D.A. (1972). "Relationship between intensity of ultrasound and induction of chromosome abnormalities". *British Journal of Radiology*, Vol. 45, pp. 320 -27.

Neilson, J.P., Munjanja, S.P. and Whitfield, C.R. (1984). "Screening for small for dates fetuses. A controlled trial". *British Medical Journal*, Vol. 289, pp. 1179-82.

Royal College of Obstetricians and Gynaecologists (R.C.O.G.). (1984). *Report of R.C.O.G. Working Party on Routine Ultrasound examination in Pregnancy*. London:R.C.O.G.

Salveson, K., Vatten Lars, J., Eik-nes, S.H. (1993). "Routine ultrasound in utero and subsequent handedness and neurological development". *British Medical Journal*, Vol. 307, pp. 159-64.

Stark, C.R., Orleans, M., Haverkamp. A.D. and Murphy, J. (1984). "Short and long term risks after exposure to diagnostic ultrasound in utero". *Obstetrics and Gynaecology*, Vol. 63, pp. 194-200.

Testart, J., Thebault, A. and Frydman, R. (1982). "Premature ovulation after ovarian ultrasonography". *British Journal of Obstetrics and Gynaecology*, Vol. 89, p. 694.

Wells, P.N.T. (1977). *Biomedical Ultrasonics.* London:Academic Press.

Wells, P.N.T. (1987a). "The prudent use of diagnostic ultrasound". *Ultrasound in Medicine and Biology*, Vol. 13, No. 7, pp. 391-400.

Wells, P.N.T. (1987b). "A Report of a British Institute of Radiology Working Group". *British Journal of Radiology,* Supplement No. 20. London:British Institute of Radiology.

Chapter 3

American Institute of Ultrasound in Medicine. (1987). In: Wells, P. (Ed). *The Safety of Diagnostic Ultrasound.* London:British Institute of Radiology.

Bakketag, L.S., Eik-Nes, S.H., Jacobsen, G., Ulsten, M.K., Brodtkorb, C.J., Balstad, P., Eriksen, B.C. and Jorgensen, N.P. (1984). "Randomised controlled trial of ultrasound screening in pregnancy". *Lancet* Vol. 2, pp. 207-11.

Bennett, M.J., Little, G., Dewhurst, C.J. and Chamberlain, G. (1982). "Predictive value of ultrasound measurements in early pregnancy. A randomised controlled trial". *British Journal of Obstetrics and Gynaecology*, Vol. 89, pp. 338-41.

British Medical Ultrasound Society (B.M.U.S.). (1984). *Safety of Diagnostic Ultrasound* . London:B.M.U.S. (Press release.)

Brock, D.J.H., Scrimgeour, J.B. and Steven, J. (1978). "Maternal alphafetoprotein screening for neural tube defects". *British Journal of Obstetrics and Gynaecology,* Vol. 85, pp. 575-81.

Bucher, N. and Schmidt, J.G. (1993). "Does routine ultrasound scanning improve outcome in pregnancy. Meta analysis of various outcome measures". *British Medical Journal,* Vol. 307, pp. 13-17.

Campbell, S. (1983). *Clinics in Obstetrics and Gynaecology.* Recent Advances, Vol. 10, No.3. London:W.B. Saunders.

Donald, I. (1974). *Clinics in Obstetrics and Gynaecology,* Vol. 10, No. 3. London:RCOG.

Eik-Nes, S.H. (1984). "Ultrasound screening in pregnancy. A randomised controlled trial". Letter Norway. *Lancet,* Vol. ii, p. 347.

Giersson, R.T. (1991). "Ultrasound instead of last menstrual period as the basis of gestational age assignment". *Ultrasound in Obstetrics and Gynaecology,* Vol.1, pp. 212-19.

Green, J. (1990). "Calming or harming". *Galton Institute Occasional Papers.* Second Series No. 2., London, pp.19-25.

Grennert, L., Persson, P.H., Gennser, G. (1978). "Benefits of ultrasound screening of a pregnant population". *Acta Obstetrica Gynaecologica Scandinavica,* Supplement, Vol. 78, pp. 5-14.

Luck, C.A. (1992). "Value of routine ultrasound scanning at 19 weeks. A four year study of 8849 deliveries". *British Medical Journal,* Vol. 304, pp. 1474-78.

MacGillivray, I. (1980). "Twins and multiple deliveries". *Clinics in Obstetrics and Gynaecology,* Vol. 7, pp. 581-600.

Neilson, J.P., Munjanja, S.P. and Whitfield, C.R. (1984). "Screening for small for dates fetuses. A controlled trial". *British Medical Journal,* Vol. 289, pp. 1179-82.

Pearce, M. J. (1987). "Making waves. Current controversies in obstetric ultrasound". *Midwifery,* Vol. 3, pp. 25-38.

Persson, P.H., Grenner, L., Gennser, G. and Kullander, S. (1979). "Improved outcome of twin pregnancies". *Acta Obstetrica Gynaecologica Scandinavica,* Vol. 58, pp. 3-12.

Pownall, M. (1987). "Just a routine matter". *Nursing Times,* Vol 83, No. 26, pp. 19-20.

Reading, A.E. and Cox, D.N. (1982). "The effects of ultrasound examination on maternal anxiety levels". *Journal of Behavioural Medicine,* Vol. 5, pp. 237-47.

Reading, A.E., Platt, L.D. (1985). "Impact of fetal testing on maternal anxiety". *Journal of Reproductive Medicine,* Vol. 30, pp. 907-10.

Reading, A.E., Cox, D.N., Campbell, S. (1988). "A controlled prospective evaluation of the acceptability of ultrasound pre-natal care". *Journal of Psychosomatic Obstetric Gynaecology,* Vol. 8, pp. 191-98.

Robinson, J. and Beech, B. (1993). "Whose risks and - - - whose benefits?". *AIMS,* Spring, Vol. 5 (1), pp. 4-6.

Royal College of Obstetrics and Gynaecology (1984). *Report of the Working Party on Routine Examination in Pregnancy.* London:RCOG.

Temmerman, M. and Buekens, P. (1991). "Cost effectiveness of routine ultrasound examination in the first trimester of pregnancy". *European Journal of Obstetrics and Gynaecology,* Vol. 39, pp. 3-6. Elsvier Science Publishers B.V. Biomedical Division 0028-2243./91/50.30.

UKCC (1991). *A Midwife's Code of Practice.* London:UKCC.

Warsof, S. L., Pearce, M. and Campbell, S. (1983). "The present place of routine ultrasound screening". *Clinics in Obstetrics and Gynaecology,* Recent Advances, Vol. 10, No. 3. W.B. Saunders, London.

Whelton, J. (1990). "Sharing the dilemmas: midwives role in pre-natal diagnosis and fetal medicine". *Professional Nurse,* Vol. 90, pp. 514-18.

Which Consumers Association. (1985). "Ultrasound in pregnancy. Should it be routine?". *Drugs and Therapeutics Bulletin,* Vol. 23, No. 15.

World Health Organisation. (1982). *Environmental Health Criteria,* 22. Geneva.

Chapter 4

Chervenak, F.A., McCullough, L.B. (1991). "Ethics an emerging subdiscipline of obstetric ultrasound, and its relevance to the routine scan". *Ultrasound in Obstetrics and Gynaecology,* Vol. 1, pp. 18-20.

Green, J., Statham, H. and Snowden, C. (1991). "Screening for fetal abnormalities; attitudes and experiences". In: Chard, T. and Richards, M.P.M. (Eds). *Benefits and Hazards of the New Obstetrics for the 1990s.* London:MacKeith Press.

Jones, D. (1978). "The need for a comprehensive counselling service for nursing students". *Journal of Advanced Nursing,* July, pp. 359-68.

Marteau, T. (1989). "Psychological costs of screening". *British Medical Journal,* Vol. 299, p. 527.

Marteau, T. (1990). "Reducing the psychological costs". *British Medical Journal,* Vol. 301, pp. 26-28.

Walkinshaw, S. (1992). "Issues in fetal medicine". Paper to Symposium. London:Galton Institute.

Wells, R. (1986). "The great conspiracy". *Nursing Times,* May, pp. 22-25.

Chapter 5

Hadlock, F.P., Harrist, R.B. and Sharman, P.S. (1985). "Estimation of fetal weight by ultrasound". *American Journal of Obstetrics and Gynaecology,* Vol. 151, pp. 333-37.

Robinson, H.P. and Fleming, J.E.E. (1975). "A critical evaluation of sonar crown-rump length measurements". *British Journal of Obstetrics and Gynaecology,* Vol. 82, pp. 702-10.

Warsof, S., Pearce, M. and Campbell, S. (1983). "The present place of routine ultrasound screening". *Clinics in Obstetric & Gynaecology.* Recent Advances, Vol. 10, No. 3. London:W.B. Saunders.

Chapter 6

Carriatore B., Stenman, U. and Ylostalo, P. (1990). "Diagnosis of ectopic pregnancy by vaginal ultrasonography, in combination with a discriminatory serum hcG level of 1000IU/I". *British Journal of Obstetrics and Gynaecology,* Vol. 97, pp. 904-8.

Goswamy, R.K. (1992). "Transvaginal ultrasonography. Useful for diagnosis." *British Medical Journal,* Vol. 304, pp.331-32.

Jolly, J. (1989a). *Missed Beginnings. Death Before Life has been Established.* London:Austen Cornish Publishers in association with The Lisa Sainsbury Foundation Series, p. 24.

Jolly, J. (1989b). *Missed Beginnings. Death Before Life has been Established.* London:Austen Cornish Publishers in association with The Lisa Sainsbury Foundation Series, p. 30.

Robinson, H.P. and Caines, J.S. (1977). "Some evidence of early pregnancy failure in patients with twin conceptions". *British Journal of Obstetrics and Gynaecology,* Vol. 84, pp. 22-25.

Tennerman, M. and Buekens, P. (1991). "Cost effectivness of routine ultrasound examination in first trimester of pregnancy". *European Journal of Obstetrics and Gynaecology and Reproductive Biology,* Vol. 39, pp. 3-6.

Varma, T.R. (1979). "Ultrasound evidence of early pregnancy failure in patients with multiple conceptions". *British Journal of Obstetrics and Gynaecology,* Vol. 86, pp. 290-92.

Chapter 7

Campbell, S. and Pearce, J. (1983). "The prenatal diagnosis of fetal structural anomalies by ultrasound. *Clinics in Obstetrics and Gynaecology,* Recent Advances, pp. 475-505. London:W.B. Saunders.

Gardosi, J. and Mongelli, M. (1993). "Risk assessment adjusted for gestational age in maternal serum screening for Down's syndrome". *British Medical Journal,* Vol. 306, pp. 1509-11.

Gowland, M. (1988). "Fetal abnormalities diagnosed from early pregnancy". *Clinical Radiology,* Vol. 39, pp.106-8.

McNay, M. (1991). "Clinical considerations in screening for fetal abnormalities". *British Medical Ultrasound Society.* Bulletin No. 63, p. 23.

Royal College of Obstetricians and Gynaecologists. (1984). *Report of the Working Party on Routine Ultrasound Examination in Pregnancy.* London:R.C.O.G.

Wald, N., Kennard, A., Densem, J., Cuckle, H., Chard, T. and Butler, L. (1992). "Ante-natal serum screening for Down's syndrome." Results of a demonstration project. *British Medical Journal,* Vol. 305, pp. 391-94.

Chapter 8

Chitty, L. and Chudleigh, T. (1993). "Choroid plexus cysts". *BMUS Bulletin,* Feb, pp. 40-41.

Lockwood, M.D., Benacerraf, M.D., Krinsky, A., Blakemore, K. *et al*. (1987). "A sonographic screening method for Down's Syndrome". *American Journal of Obstetrics and Gynaecology,* Vol. 157, pp. 803-8.

Twining, P. (1993). "Choroid plexus cysts: a conservative approach". *BMUS Bulletin,* Feb., p. 43.

Walkinshaw, S.A. (1993). "Isolated choroid plexus cysts". *BMUS Bulletin,* Feb., p. 39.

Warsof, S., Pearce, J.M. and Campbell, S. (1983). "The present place of routine ultrasound screening". *Clinics in Obstetrics and Gynaecology,* Vol. 10, No. 3. London:RCOG.

Chapter 9

Allan, L.D., Crawford, D.C., Chita, S.K. and Tynan, M.J. (1986). "Prenatal screening for congenital heart disease". *British Medical Journal,* Vol. 292, pp.1717-19.

Fowlie, A. (1991). "Ultrasound examination of the chest and abdomen". *BMUS Bulletin,* No. 63, Nov., pp.37-40.

Gibbon, W. and Hayward, C. (1991). "The role of ultrasound in the management of renal tract anomalies detected antenatally". *BMUS Bulletin,* No. 63, pp. 14-15.

Chapter 10

Anthony, R., Bringle, R. and Kinney, K. (1984). *Psychological Aspects of Genetic Counselling.* Edited by Emery, A.E.H. and Pullen, pp. 75-94. London:Academic Press.

Kenyon, S. (1988). "Support after termination for fetal abnormality". *Midwives Chronicle and Nursing Notes,* Vol. 101, No.1, 205, p. 190.

Twining, P. (1991). "The ultrasound markers of chromosome disease". *BMUS Bulletin,* Nov, pp. 30-34.

Chapter 11

Barker, P. (1993). *"Fetal Origins of Infant and Adult Disease."* London:BMJ Publishing Group.

Chudleigh, P. and Pearce, M. (1983). "The placenta". In: *Obstetric Ultrasound. How, Why, and When.* p.125. London:Churchill Livingstone.

Fitzhardinge, P.M. and Steven, E.M. (1972). "The small for dates infant. 11 Neurological and intellectual sequelae". *Paediatrics,* Vol. 49, p. 50.

Lin, C.C., Moanad, A.M., Rosecrow, P.J. and River, P. (1980). "Acid base characteristics of fetuses with intra-uterine growth retardation during labor and delivery". *American Journal of Obstetrics and Gynecology,* Vol. 137, p. 553.

Manning, F.A., Platt, L.D. and Sipos, L. (1980). "Antepartum fetal evaluation; development of fetal biophysical profile". *American Journal of Obstetrics and Gynaecology,* Vol. 136, pp. 787-95.

Pearce, J.M. and Campbell, S. (1983). "Ultrasonic monitoring of normal and abnormal fetal growth". In: Laurenson, N.R. (Ed). *Principals and modern management of high risk pregnancy.* New York:Plenum, pp. 57-100.

Proud, J. and Grant, A. (1987). "Third trimester grading by placental ultrasonography as a test of fetal wellbeing". *British Medical Journal,* Vol. 294, pp. 1641-44.

Usher, P. and Mclean, M. (1974). "Normal fetal growth and the significance of fetal growth retardation". In: Davis, J. and Dobbing, (Eds). *Scientific Foundations of Paediatrics.* London William Heineman, pp. 69-80.

Wilcox, M., Gardosi, J., Mongelli, M., Ray, C. and Johnson, I. (1993). "Birth weight from pregnancies dated by ultrasonography in a multicultural British population". *British Medical Journal,* pp. 307.

Chapter 12

Nicolaides, K.H., Bilardo, C.M., Soothill, P.W. and Campbell, S. (1988). *British Medical Journal,* Vol. 297, pp. 1026-27.

Satomura, A. (1959). "Study of flow patterns in peripheral arteries by ultrasonics". *Journal of the Acoustical Society of Japan,* Vol. 15, p. 151.

Trudinger, B.J., Giles, W.B. and Cook, R.N. (1985). "Flow velocity waveforms in the maternal uteroplacental and fetal umbilical placental circulations". *British Journal of Obstetrics and Gynaecology,* Vol. 152, No. 2, p. 152.

Tyrell, S.N., Lilford, R.J., MacDonald N.E.J., Porter, J. and Gupta, J.K. (1990). "Randomised comparison of routine vs highly selective use of Doppler ultrasound and biophysical scoring to investigate high risk pregnancies". *British Journal of Obstetrics and Gynaecology,* Vol. 97, pp. 909-16.

Tyrell, S., Mason, G.C., Lilford, R.J. and Porter, J. (1993). "Randomised comparison of routine versus highly selective use of Doppler ultrasound in low risk pregnancies". *British Journal of Obstetrics and Gynaecology,* Vol. 100, pp.130-33.

Chapter 13

Dornan, J.C. (1993). "Early amniocentesis". *British Medical Ultrasound Bulletin,* Vol. 1, No. 3, pp. 34-35.

Jennett, B. (1984). "High technology medicine". Nuffield Provincial Hospitals Trust. London, pp. 133-34.

Maxwell, D., Johnson, P., Hurley, P., Neales, K., Allan, L. and Knott, P. (1991). "Fetal blood sampling; an evaluation of pregnancy loss in relation to indication". *British Journal Obstetrics and Gynaecology,* Vol. pp. 265-73.

Medical Research Council. (1991). "European trial of chorionic villus sampling and amniocentesis. *Lancet,* Vol. 1, pp. 1491-99.

Tabor, A., Philip, J., Madsen, M., Bang, J., Obel, E. and Norgaard-Pederson, B. (1986). "Randomised controlled trial of genetic amniocentesis in 4,606 low risk women". *Lancet,* Vol. 1, p. 1267.

Index

T

U

V

W

Y